UK Ambulance Services
Emergency Response
Driver's Handbook

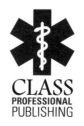

CLASS
PROFESSIONAL
PUBLISHING

Disclaimer
The Association of Ambulance Chief Executives has made every effort to ensure that the information and diagrams contained in this handbook are accurate at the time of publication. However, the handbook cannot always contain all the information necessary for determining appropriate action and cannot address all individual situations; therefore, individuals using this book must ensure they have the appropriate knowledge and skills to enable suitable interpretation.

The Association of Ambulance Chief Executives does not guarantee, and accepts no legal liability of whatever nature arising from or connected to, the accuracy, reliability, currency or completeness of the content of this handbook.

Users of this handbook must always be aware that innovations or alterations after the date of publication may not be incorporated in the content. As part of its commitment to defining national standards, the Association will periodically issue updates to the content and users should ensure that they are using the most up-to-date version. Please note, however, that the Association of Ambulance Chief Executives assumes no responsibility whatsoever for the content of external resources.

It is recognised that a number of the laws in NI and Scotland differ somewhat from the laws throughout the rest of the UK; if operating in these areas then reference to these laws must be made.

Printing history
First published 2012
This second edition published 2014

The author and publisher welcome feedback from the users of this book.
Please contact the publisher:
Class Professional Publishing,
The Exchange, Express Park, Bristol Road, Bridgwater, TA6 4RR, UK.
Telephone: 01278 427800
Email: post@class.co.uk
Website: www.classprofessional.co.uk

Class Professional Publishing is an imprint of Class Publishing Ltd.

A CIP catalogue record for this book is available from the British Library.

ISBN 978 185959 435 3 (paperback, 2nd edition)
ISBN 978 185959 436 0 (ebook, 2nd edition)

Designed and typeset by Typematter

Cover photograph supplied courtesy of London Ambulance Service NHS Trust

Line illustrations by David Woodroffe

Printed in Slovenia by arrangement with KINT Ljubljana

Contents

Foreword

This second and revised edition of the *UK Ambulance Services Emergency Response Driver's Handbook* is designed for ambulance personnel undertaking NHS Ambulance Service emergency response driver training and education programmes. It also contains generic and relevant information that can serve as guidance and advice for drivers in non-emergency roles.

It is intended to enhance the practical instruction delivered by appropriately qualified instructors by providing a reference that can be used for self-study, either before or during a course, and for ready reference post-training to maintain and further develop your skills and competencies in emergency response driving.

Certain changes are taking place relating to the legal framework surrounding emergency response driving (for example, Section 19 of the Road Safety Act 2006) and this second and revised edition has been written in anticipation (where possible) of these legislative changes and to reflect current best practice.

It is the responsibility of the driver of any vehicle to understand and comply with current legislation. Where legislation applies to NHS vehicles or more generally to 'ambulances', it is important that any differences are understood.

Paul Jones-Roberts
Chair of Driver Training Advisory Group (DTAG)
On behalf of the NHS Ambulance Services

Acknowledgements

This handbook and the previous edition were initiated by the Driver Training Advisory Group (DTAG) and endorsed by the Association of Ambulance Chief Executives (AACE), who recommend that it is used for driver instruction and education. The handbook was produced in consultation with UK NHS ambulance driver training leads. In addition to this, recognition and appreciation is made to Mr Owain Davies for his contributions to this manual.

Acknowledgements to the DTAG members of:

- East Midlands Ambulance Service NHS Trust
- East of England Ambulance Service NHS Trust
- London Ambulance Service NHS Trust
- NHS Isle of Wight Ambulance Service
- North East Ambulance Service NHS Foundation Trust
- North West Ambulance Service NHS Trust
- Northern Ireland Ambulance Service Health and Social Care Trust
- Scottish Ambulance Service
- South Central Ambulance Service NHS Foundation Trust
- South East Coast Ambulance Service NHS Foundation Trust
- South Western Ambulance Service NHS Foundation Trust
- Welsh Ambulance Service NHS Trust
- West Midlands Ambulance Service NHS Foundation Trust
- Yorkshire Ambulance Service NHS Trust

Appreciation is also given to the DTAG editorial sub-group who undertook the review in preparation for this second edition, in particular Paul Jones-Roberts (NWAS), Mike Dunford (SCAS), Robin Gwinnett (SWAST) and Simon Macartney (SECAmb).

Introduction

This manual has been designed as a training reference to assist drivers of emergency ambulance vehicles. It will help them to understand the standards and practices that aim to provide maximum protection to crews, passengers and other road users. It is not intended to be an exhaustive guide and should be used in conjunction with the current editions of *Roadcraft: The Police Driver's Handbook* and *The Highway Code*.

The book makes it clear that technical mastery alone is not enough to ensure that drivers are safe; they also have to have a sound knowledge of legislation, of the current editions of *The Highway Code* and *Roadcraft: The Police Driver's Handbook*, and of road traffic law relating to the exemptions and non-exemptions applied to emergency response driving. This will equip them with the ability to modify their driving style in response to prevailing road conditions and any other hazards that may present themselves, in order to reach their destination as quickly, and as safely, as possible.

One of the main aims of this book is to minimise operational road risk and reduce undue public concern about incidents involving emergency vehicles responding to emergency calls. There are now increased possibilities for legal proceedings where there is evidence of unsafe, dangerous or careless driving, as determined by the Road Traffic Act 1988.

No circumstances can justify endangering lives and/or property by breaking the law, whether the action is exempt or not. No emergency, no matter how serious, will justify causing an accident, especially as mitigating circumstances may be negated. Emergency vehicles being driven in any situation will attract attention and, in some cases, public criticism – particularly when using emergency warning equipment. Great care and attention should be given to the manner in which you drive a service vehicle in order to minimise any such criticism.

Although the title of this book suggests that it is focused only on emergency response driving, it also aims to provide advice and guidance to drivers of non-emergency vehicles, for example patient-transport service drivers.

1 The Law in Relation to Ambulance Driving

All road users are subject to the rules of the road and the laws in relation to driving, including *The Highway Code*, the Road Traffic Act 1988 and the Road Safety Act 2006. As well as being fully conversant with these, drivers of emergency vehicles must also understand and comply with additional legislation relating to high-speed driving (s19 RSA 2006 when enacted), driving licences and their medical fitness to drive.

Ambulance drivers must also comply with the policies of their individual NHS Trust or organisation regarding driving licence checks and their road traffic collision reporting and incident reporting procedures.

Learning outcomes

By the end of this chapter you should:

▲ Understand the importance of adhering to the principles of *The Highway Code*.

▲ Know your responsibilities to drive in a manner that does not constitute 'dangerous', 'careless' or 'inconsiderate' driving or parking.

▲ Know your obligations under civil law.

▲ Understand who is legally authorised to claim the exemption of speed according to Section 19 of the Road Safety Act 2006.

▲ Know the importance of following your Trust's procedural requirements regarding motor vehicle insurance.

▲ Understand the DVLA's medical standards that must be met for different categories of driving licence, and the requirement to comply with your Trust's driving licence checks.

▲ Know the importance and legal requirements of following your Trust's road traffic collision and incident-reporting procedures.

General driving guidelines

The Highway Code outlines the rules and guidelines that promote road safety in the UK. It is produced by HM Stationery Office in a number of formats and available to view free online. While failure to observe advice within *The Highway Code* does not render that person liable to criminal proceedings, the Road Traffic Act 1988 (The Road Traffic (NI) Order 2007) says that any failure to adhere to the Code's principles can be used to establish or negate liability in civil or criminal proceedings.

All NHS Ambulance Trust drivers should have a sound knowledge of *The Highway Code*. It is a statutory obligation for all staff to drive in accordance with current road traffic legislation, which means that it is the responsibility of drivers to maintain their knowledge of the current edition of *The Highway Code*. You should always drive in a manner that demonstrates your skill and knowledge of driving matters to other road users in relation to the *Code*.

> **REMEMBER!**
> It is the responsibility of drivers to maintain their knowledge of the current edition of *The Highway Code*.

Driving standards required by law

If a person drives a mechanically propelled vehicle on a road or other public place without due care and attention, or without reasonable consideration for other persons using the road or place, he is guilty of an offence.

(Road Traffic Act 1988, amended 1991)

Civil law

General rules, techniques and advice for all drivers and riders are contained within the current version of *The Highway Code*.

In addition to this, legislative changes that are expected to be enacted during 2014 will impose certain criteria on who is legally authorised to claim the exemption of speed. When enacted, Section 19 of the Road Safety Act 2006 is likely to determine that only drivers who have satisfactorily completed a course of training in driving vehicles at high speed will be legally permitted to claim the exemption of exceeding speed limits. In addition, they must be able to demonstrate compliance with the proposed competencies as specified in the Codes of Practice (COP) 'driver competencies'. This is also the case for instructors responsible for the delivery of this training, who must satisfy the COP and the 'instructor competencies', which determine that the undertaking of this training must be carried out by appropriately qualified instructors.

It will be a requirement that driver competencies are assessed at intervals not exceeding five years.

Reference for the above is:

DfT Speed Limit Exemptions: Consultation document
https://www.gov.uk/government/uploads/system/uploads/attachment_data/file/16261/consultation-document.pdf

Sentences for dangerous driving

In 2003 the Court of Appeal issued guideline penalties that should be considered when an incident results in death by dangerous driving. The Lord Chief Justice said that, while jail terms should only be imposed where necessary: 'normally the only appropriate sentence to an offender found guilty of these offences is a custodial sentence'.

The Court of Appeal stated that, when determining the appropriate sentence, courts should bear in mind: 'how important it is to drive home the message that dangerous driving has a potentially horrific impact'.

In a summary, the three judges said: 'Drivers must know that, if a person is killed as a result of their driving dangerously, a custodial sentence will normally be imposed no matter what the mitigating circumstances.'

This applies to all road users equally. No emergency, no matter how serious, will justify you being involved in an accident.

Motor insurance

NHS Trust employees **must** inform their own insurer of any road traffic collisions that they are involved in, or motoring convictions received while driving during their work activities for the Trust. In addition you must inform your own insurer of any motoring convictions received while driving Trust vehicles. Failure to do so may result in your insurance being declared void by your insurers as you will have failed to disclose your full driving history.

If you receive penalty points or convictions while not at work, you should inform your employer as per local guidelines.

Collisions involving ambulances

In the IAM published research called *Licensed to Skill: Contributory Factors in Road Accidents*, the Institute of Advanced Motorists analysed more than 700,000 road accidents that happened between 2005 and 2009 in Great Britain. Thankfully, 'emergency vehicles on call' were only cited as a contributory factor in 0.3% of fatal accidents.

However, as there are no clearly published statistics for the UK, the actual level of risk is poorly described and reliable data on accident rates is hard to find.

There are, however, reports that one large metropolitan ambulance service experienced involvement in more than four collisions a day, ranging from minor collisions to serious incidents, and in one year this meant total costs of £2.6 million, including £586,000 for repairs and more than £2 million in legal fees.

Licence categories C1 & D1

Most NHS Ambulance Trusts operate category C1 vehicles (which weigh between 3,500kg and 7,500kg) and category D1 vehicles (with 9 to 16 passenger seats).

The Driver and Vehicle Licensing Agency (DVLA) specify medical standards for different groups of drivers:

- **Group 1** – drivers of motor cars and motorcycles.

- **Group 2** – drivers of category C large goods vehicles (LGV), for example lorries; and category D passenger carrying vehicles (PCV), for example buses.

These categories are either held by individuals under implied rights or are attained through licence acquisition by way of theory and practical tests depending on the year the learner driving test was passed.

Drivers who obtained entitlement to Group 1 category B (motor car) before 1 January 1997 have an entitlement to category C1 and D1. Holders of C1 and D1 entitlement retain this entitlement until their licence expires or is medically revoked. On renewal, the higher medical standards required for Group 2 will apply.

The information below is taken from the Gov.uk website. Legislation regarding driver licensing is often reviewed, and changes and amendments could be made. It is vitally important that you keep yourself up to date with any potential changes.

C1 & D1 drivers passing a driving test after 19 January 2013

If you passed your driving test in categories C, CE, C1, C1E, D, DE, D1 or D1E after 19 January 2013, you will get a licence valid for five years.

You will need to sign a declaration to show that you still meet the medical standards every five years up to the age of 45.

After age 45, you will need to provide a medical examination report every five years to renew your driving entitlement.

C1 & D1 drivers who passed a driving test before 19 January 2013

Drivers under 45 years old

If you passed a driving test in categories C, CE, C1, C1E, D, DE, D1 or D1E, you will come under the new rules when you renew your driving licence.

When you renew your licence you will receive a new one valid for five years. Every time you renew you will need to confirm that you still meet the medical standards.

If you apply to replace your licence because it has been lost or stolen, or your personal details have changed, your new licence will run until the end of your original period.

However, if you update your photo at the same time, you will come under the new five-year rule.

Drivers over 45 years old

Drivers over 45 years of age will continue to renew their entitlement as they do now. When you renew your licence at the end of a five-year period, you will need to provide a medical examination report.

More information can be found on the DVLA website.

Medical fitness to drive

The additional legal responsibilities that drivers must comply with relating to medical fitness to drive are specified in the DVLA's Drivers Medical Group publication *Medical Standards of Fitness to Drive*, which is updated regularly and can be found on the DVLA website.

Driving licence checks

Ambulance services have a duty to check the driving licences of all staff that drive service vehicles. These checks take place on a regular basis, normally annually (refer to local procedures).

It is the individual licence holder's responsibility to ensure that their driving licence is valid and in date. Photo card driving licences are only valid for ten years – section 4b on the photo card provides the expiry date. The DVLA issues reminders for this.

Road traffic collision reporting and incident-reporting procedures

Each ambulance service has individual procedures in place for reporting incidents involving motor vehicles. Drivers of service vehicles should ensure full compliance with local procedures and, above all, be fully conversant with the legal requirements of being involved in an accident as per Section 170 of the Road Traffic Act 1988.

Knowledge recap questions

1. How frequently should driver competencies in driving at high speed be assessed according to Section 19 of the Road Safety Act 2006?

2. Why is it necessary to inform your own insurer of any road traffic collision that you are involved in while driving an emergency response vehicle for your Trust?

3. You have to sign a declaration to show that you still meet the required medical standards when your C1 and D1 driving licence is renewed. How does this change when you reach the age of 45?

4. Whose responsibility is it to ensure that your driving licence is valid and in date?

2 Legal Exemptions and Non-Exemptions

Due to the nature of their work, emergency ambulance vehicles are exposed to hazardous activities on a regular basis. The urgency of their purpose provides for certain exemptions to driving law; however, these exemptions can only be claimed if the driver's actions can be justified.

This chapter offers advice and guidance in relation to the claiming of specific legal exemptions and identifies exemptions that cannot be claimed (non-exemptions).

Learning outcomes

By the end of this chapter you should:

▲ Understand the specific circumstances in which emergency vehicle drivers are exempt from various requirements of road traffic legislation.

▲ Be aware that some exemptions apply when dealing with any category of patient but others may only be claimed while engaged on emergencies.

▲ Understand that legal exemptions do not include driving without due care and attention or driving at speed in a manner that is dangerous.

▲ Know that traffic law non-exemptions apply even when driving under emergency conditions.

Legal exemptions

Ambulance Service drivers can claim exemptions to road traffic law when justifiable and when the vehicle is being used for ambulance purposes. You may be liable to prosecution unless you can demonstrate that you can satisfy the above criteria.

When claiming exemptions the following statement MUST apply in all cases:

*The exemption can be claimed **if the observance of that provision would be likely to hinder the use of the vehicle for the purpose for which it is being used on that occasion.***

The driver and the Trust are obliged, under the Corporate Manslaughter and Homicide Act 2007 and the Road Safety Act 2006, to afford, at all times, the maximum protection to other road users.

The following section offers advice and guidance in relation to the claiming of specific legal exemptions.

- The statutory speed limit can be exceeded, but only if it is safe to do so. *s.87 Road Traffic Regulation Act 1984 (speed)*

- Static, portable and inoperative traffic lights can be treated as a give way. *Regulation 36(1)(b) The Traffic Signs Regulations & General Directions 2002 (red light)*

- Vehicles may pass on the wrong side of keep left/right signs if progress is likely to be hindered, no danger is caused to other vehicles, and it can be justified that there were no other alternatives (in exceptional circumstances). *Regulation 15(2) The Traffic Signs Regulations & General Directions 2002*

REMEMBER!

While exempt from adhering to speed limits, there is still a statutory requirement to maintain safety and to offer the maximum protection to other road users – legal exemptions do not include driving without due care and attention or driving at speed in a manner that is dangerous.

Road traffic law exemptions that apply when dealing with any category of patient

Stopping on clearways

s.5 Road Traffic Regulation Act 1984

- Always ensure that you have the correct personal protective equipment (PPE) on when exiting the vehicle on fast-flowing roads.

Parking within the zigzag area of a pedestrian crossing

Regulation 27(3)(c) Traffic Signs Regulations & General Directions 2002

Remember the following points:

- Increased risk to pedestrians
- Scene safety is paramount
- Where possible ensure police/traffic control assistance.

Parking within areas controlled by double white/yellow (or red) lines

Regulation 26(5)(b) Traffic Signs Regulations & General Directions 2002

Remember the following points:

- Consideration of road layout to minimise risks
- Assessment of patient condition and mobility
- Keep parking time to a minimum.

Leaving the engine running while parked

Regulation 107 Road Vehicles (Construction and Use) Regulations 1986

Remember the following points:

- Vehicle security/use of 'run lock'
- Heating and lighting factors
- Environmental factors.

Parking on the offside of the road at night

Regulation 101 Road Vehicles (Construction and Use) Regulations 1986
Regulation 24 Road Vehicle Lighting Regulations 1989

Remember the following points:

- Headlights off
- Leave sidelights on
- Use hazard warning lights (if causing a temporary obstruction to traffic)
- Use of personal protective equipment (PPE).

Parking on a footway/verge/central reservation

s.5 Road Traffic Regulation Act 1984 & s16(d) Motorways Traffic England and Wales) Regulations 1982
By-laws

Remember the following points:

- Obstruction to pedestrians
- Hazard of soft verges
- Footpath and vehicle damage.

Road traffic law exemptions that apply only while engaged on emergencies

Exceeding statutory speed limits

s.87(1)(2) Road Traffic Regulation Act 1984 (Amended 2006)

Remember the following points:

- Danger of 'red mist' affecting driver
- Unpredictability of other road users
- Traffic calming measures in place
- Suggested 20mph maximum increase above speed limit.

- Increased rate of hazard prioritisation necessary
- Greater density of hazards = reduce speed
- Weather conditions
- Be aware of the limitations of the vehicle and the driver.

Choosing an appropriate speed

When responding under emergency driving conditions the overriding consideration is safety. You must always be able to stop safely in the distance you can see to be clear. Your Ambulance Trust or Service may have policy relating to the use of speed exemptions and you should adhere to these at all times. See Appendix 5, Speed and safety.

Road traffic and weather conditions should also be taken into consideration when deciding on an appropriate speed to make progress.

Red mist

This term is used to describe a psychological state that can arise when drivers of emergency response vehicles are travelling at speed, focusing on what may be presented at the incident they are travelling to rather than their driving. It can cloud one's ability to assess driving risks realistically and to make the logical decision essential for the safety of the crew and other road users.

Treating a red traffic light as a give way – includes zebra crossings (not traffic controlled)

Regulations 33, 34, 35, 36(1)(a), 38(a/b) Traffic Signs Regulations & General Directions 2002 Motorway
Regulations 47, 48, 49 Traffic Signs Regulations & General Directions 2002

Remember the following points:

- Never attempt to force other road users into illegal manoeuvres
- Always give precedence to pedestrians showing an intention to use the crossing
- Restrained approach with maximum use of warning equipment
- Are all road users aware of the emergency vehicle?
- Use vehicle positioning on approach to indicate intended route
- Possibility of another emergency vehicle on an opposing route
- Adjust the speed of your approach to anticipate traffic lights changing to green
- Where no progress can be made, the ambulance should adopt a 'hold back' position and turn audible warnings off, to prevent traffic moving through the red light (this is sometimes referred to as **effective non-use**).

Pedestrian crossings

Drivers must give precedence to any pedestrians crossing the road who are on the part of the carriageway that lies within the limits of the crossing or on a central reservation lying between two crossings that does not form part of a system of staggered crossings.

Do not proceed in a manner or at a time that is likely to endanger any pedestrians or vehicles approaching or waiting at the crossing. Do not cause the driver of any such vehicles to change their speed or direction in order to avoid an accident.

Use of audible warnings at night
Regulation 99 Road Vehicles (Construction and Use) Regulations 1986

Remember the following points:

- Determine the need for an advanced audible warning
- Level of traffic/pedestrian activity
- Consider other audible devices/duration
- Remember siren off = speed off
- Intelligent use of sirens – non-use must be justified; you must use them if their use would help or warn others.

Observing keep left/right signs
Regulation 15(2) Traffic Signs Regulations & General Directions 2002

Remember the following points:

- Dangers of returning to the nearside
- Essential use of mirrors and signals
- Hazards of central barrier/separate carriageway
- Roundabout entry and direction of travel
- Oncoming traffic
- Pedestrians may only look one way
- Maximum use of audible/visual warnings
- Speed reduction.

Motorway regulations (where you need to do so in order to avoid or prevent an accident, or to obtain or give the help required at an accident scene)
Motorways Traffic (England and Wales) Regulations 1982

Remember the following points:

- Higher speeds/density of traffic

- Essential use of PPE and visual warnings

- Increased engine/road noise masks sirens

- Use of hard shoulder running

- Parking under police or other supervision

- Situation if first vehicle on scene.

Some areas have introduced a system called 'Smart Motorways' or 'all-lane running' which uses technology to help relieve congestion and make journey times more reliable. This includes controlling speeds to improve traffic flow and providing better information to drivers on overhead signs. Most recognisably the hard shoulder can be converted to a traffic lane at peak times, or permanently, with emergency refuge areas. This extra lane creates vital additional capacity with no worsening of safety. You should therefore consult local policies and procedures for attending incidents in these areas.

Entering a bus lane during its hours of operation

By-laws (possible local operator policy variance for non-emergency and use of contraflow bus lanes)

Remember the following points:

- In emergencies, traffic usually pulls over to the left, but foreign vehicles may inadvertently move right

- Parked cars during non-operation times

- Check the hours of operation

- Bus lane/street may have shared occupancy

- Proximity of pedestrians

- Avoid contraflow bus lanes.

Entering a pedestrian precinct
Traffic Signs Regulations & General Directions 2002
By-laws

Remember the following points:

- Speed of entry into precinct
- Speed of negotiation = extreme caution
- Conform to direction of traffic flow
- The siren might not be the most suitable audible warning – consider using the vehicle horn
- Give pedestrians precedence
- Security of vehicle when parked
- Danger of being blocked in by delivery vehicles, etc.

Roadworks

There are occasions when roads are restricted to single-lane traffic flow and managed by either a convoy vehicle or a road worker operating a stop-and-go board. On the approach to these hazards, all emergency warning equipment (EWE) should be activated to alert the workers of your approach. Having arrived at the area of work, the vehicle should be brought to a halt with sirens deactivated until it is indicated by the workers managing the traffic that it is safe to proceed.

Non-exemptions

These conditions apply even when driving under emergency conditions. No driver is exempt from driving or parking in a manner that is dangerous, careless or inconsiderate and that may put either lives or property at risk.

Drivers of emergency response vehicles cannot claim exemptions for the following actions:

1. Dangerous driving

2. Dangerous parking

3. Careless driving

4. Failure to stop if involved in a road traffic collision

5. Driving without wearing a seat belt other than when stated in *The Highway Code*

6. Failure to obey a red traffic signal controlling a fire station or railway level crossing

7. Crossing or straddling a solid white line, nearest to you, along the centre of the road when not entitled to do so subject to rule 129 of *The Highway Code*

   This means you MUST NOT cross or straddle the white line unless it is safe and you need to enter adjoining premises or a side road. You may cross the line if necessary, providing the road is clear, to pass a stationary vehicle, or overtake a pedal cycle, horse or road maintenance vehicle, if they are travelling at 10mph [16km/h] or less. Or if instructed to do so by a police officer in uniform.

   s.36 Road Traffic Act 1988

   Regulations 10 and 26 Traffic Signs Regulations & General Directions 2002

8. Failing to obey a one-way traffic sign

9. Failing to obey a no entry sign

10. Failing to obey a stop or give way sign

11. Failing to obey any other instructional sign, such as no right turn.

Knowledge recap questions

1. Name two road traffic law exemptions that apply when dealing with any category of patient.

2. Name two road traffic law exemptions that only apply when dealing with an emergency response situation.

3. State three safety factors that should be kept in mind when exceeding statutory speed limits.

4. Describe how best to approach a pedestrian crossing when driving under emergency response conditions?

5. Do traffic law non-exemptions apply when driving under emergency conditions?

6. Explain the procedure that should be followed when roadworks are encountered while driving under blue light conditions?

7. Name two road traffic law non-exemptions.

3 Driver Characteristics and Responsibilities

It is well known that human factors are a significant contributing factor to most road traffic collisions. Emergency response drivers need to demonstrate the highest standards and must be appropriately trained to deal with these human factors when driving under emergency conditions.

This chapter considers some of the skills and behaviours essential for an emergency response driver as well as the stress factors that can impact on how drivers carry out their duties. It also covers drivers' responsibilities for ensuring the comfort of their passengers.

Learning outcomes

By the end of this chapter you should:

▲ Know the specialist skills required by emergency response drivers.

▲ Understand how driver attitudes and behaviour can contribute to increased risk.

▲ Recognise how intrusive thoughts can influence the decision-making process.

▲ Recognise the different operational driving stress factors that may impact on emergency response drivers and how their effects can be combated.

▲ Recognise how passenger comfort can be compromised and the driver's responsibility to prevent this.

Driving skills

There are a number of important specialist elements in emergency vehicle driving. Drivers should possess the ability to:

- Deal with several complicated tasks simultaneously and to a high standard

- Spread their attention during a difficult drive to be able to deal with it in a systematic way

- Build up awareness of the whole environment

- Plan accurately and quickly

- Anticipate based on observations and experience

- Make sound judgements in all circumstances

- Remain alert and vigilant to ensure no hazard is overlooked.

As there is no predetermined procedure for every conceivable type of situation that develops, drivers must continually perform a dynamic risk assessment on the changing environment and conditions.

You must be fully aware that attitudes related to driving under emergency response conditions are influenced considerably by reduced concentration and intrusive thoughts, however insignificant they may seem (such as focusing on the potential incident that is being responded to, personal influences relating to work, private life or fatigue), which compromise the decision-making process.

A robust driving response system needs to be employed to help equip the driver with the ability to perform safely regardless of outside influences. You must bear in mind that you may be liable to prosecution if your driving falls below a safe standard. Driving commentary is an effective tool to help develop situational awareness, anticipation planning and preparation (see Appendix 4).

The NHS fleet

The diverse range of vehicles in the NHS operational fleet will sometimes determine the necessity for additional training or even the requirement to hold certain driving licence categories. Regardless of the vehicle type, any driver responsible for a vehicle must ensure that they are appropriately trained and equipped to operate it, that they are fully conversant with the vehicle controls by performing a pre-driving check and that they are satisfied that the vehicle is legally roadworthy by performing a vehicle daily inspection (see Chapter 4).

There has been some interesting research on how different types of emergency drivers are affected by different sources of stress (Sharp *et al*, 1997; Dorn, 2013). Three types were identified:

● Those for whom personal reward is the most important factor, such as salary, fringe benefits, job security and working conditions

● Those who are people orientated, where helping the public, providing a service and working with people is most important

● Those for whom a professional career is most important, valuing the high prestige, independence and use of professional skills required by the job.

Further reading

A more detailed discussion on the topic of attitudes and driver behaviour can be found in *Roadcraft* and other publications on the subject by Dr Lisa Dorn of Cranfield University and Dr Gordon Sharp, author of *Human Aspects of Police Driving*.

Operational driving stress

There is evidence to show that those who are repeatedly exposed to stress can be more accident prone. The most useful definition of stress is: 'the perception by the driver of the demands placed on him or her and their ability to cope with these demands'. The following categories have been identified as types of operational stress that emergency service drivers may be exposed to.

Key term

Operational driving stress – the perception by the driver of the demands placed on him or her and their ability to cope with these demands.

Anticipatory responses

These can vary from person to person and cover feelings such as pre-examination nerves and physical symptoms such as mild gastric irritation, nausea and even vomiting. These symptoms can occur for some period of time before an event and may or may not subside when the event is taking place.

Alarm reaction

This is the reaction set off by an alarm, similar to an athlete on the starting line, and is experienced by anyone about to be involved in a drive that requires full concentration and maximum effort. Symptoms can include a dry mouth, sweaty palms and a pounding heart. This heightened level of awareness enables a better performance provided it does not become too intense.

Task-related stress

This can manifest itself during a task, when there are difficulties getting to an incident, the driver is unaware of the full details of the incident, or there is anxiety over the actions that are required upon arrival.

'Overloading' induced by task-related stress can lead to:

- Omissions by failing to respond to stimuli

- Errors where the incorrect action is taken

- Approximation wherein quality drops, which may cause danger

- 'Coning' of attention, where concentration is focused on one narrow aspect and the driver can miss important hazards.

Life-threatening stress

Under the extreme pressure of time-sensitive responses and other similar activities, stress can cause the brain to close down all but those actions it considers are required to preserve life. This can result in rigid muscle tension, where the person freezes and is unable to take actions to save themselves, or blind panic, where actions are taken without any reason.

Cumulative incident stress

In dealing with distressing incidents, the brain can eventually block out some of the distressing aspects. This can result in a lack of correct information gathering.

Post-error dwell reaction

This is another mild stress reaction that can occur when a person carries out an inappropriate action or makes an error. The person dwells on the action that has happened instead of concentrating on the matter now in hand.

Work-related stress

Work stresses can have an important bearing on operational stress reactions. They can include dealing with mundane tasks, feelings of career stagnation or uncertainty, unpopular work schedules and deteriorating working relationships.

The reactions to this type of stress may include: apathy, boredom, difficulty making decisions, feelings of a life of crises, frustration, headaches, impatience, indigestion, insomnia, irritability, nausea, sweating and feelings that work is becoming harder.

Combating the effects of stress

The first line of defence is to recognise the factors that cause stress; the second is to rely on training. Stress can be combated using the following measures (Sharp *et al*, 1997):

- Using all mental capacity available; tasks that have been learnt are more likely to be remembered

- Maintaining a high level of general health

- Learning to relax

- Approaching driving in a calm, confident manner, using the skills that have been learnt

- Trying to share difficult decision making as a team

- Keeping problems separate from operational driving

- Not allowing previous incidents to cloud your judgement

- Putting minor errors to one side

- Learning to recognise stresses and adjust.

Professional support

There are many ways to deal with these stresses. Some people may be able to employ their own coping strategies; however, anyone experiencing difficulties should obtain professional help from the various agencies that are available.

Drivers' responsibility to ensure passenger comfort

Regardless of the type of driving being undertaken – whether emergency response driving (ERD) or non-response – the driver of an ambulance vehicle has a responsibility to ensure that patients' and passengers' journeys are smooth and comfortable as well as safe.

It is important to remember that a patient's medical condition can affect their comfort during a journey and also that a lack of consideration could possibly exacerbate that condition. Therefore, driving plans need to be developed to take this into account.

REMEMBER!

A patient's medical condition can greatly affect their comfort during a journey. In cases of traumatic injury, the prognosis can be significantly influenced by the smoothness (or lack of) of their journey. The patient's needs must be considered and facilitated for during the formulation of driving plans.

As an example, a patient who has sustained a fracture or is suffering from rheumatoid arthritis will be particularly susceptible to discomfort from uneven road surfaces or potholes. There are other traumatic injury types whereby poor acceleration sense, harsh braking or cornering can significantly influence the patient's prognosis.

It can be a daunting experience for anyone travelling in the saloon of an ambulance; this is exacerbated by the lack of vision afforded, which does not allow for the anticipation of vehicle movements as it could when travelling in a car.

It is therefore important that the drive is smooth and the system of vehicle control is applied effectively, with emphasis given to good acceleration sense, early braking for hazards and the execution of tapered braking.

Vary the brake pressure when bringing the vehicle to a stop, to avoid unnecessary jolting, by:

1. Gently taking up the free play in the pedal.
2. Increasing the brake pressure progressively as required to bring the vehicle to a halt.
3. Relaxing pedal pressure as unwanted road speed is lost.
4. Releasing the pedal just before stopping to avoid jerking.

While engaged on ERD it is useful to inform the attendant of approaching hazards that may affect vehicle movements so that they can ensure that they are safely restrained or suitably positioned.

When loading patients, consider the seating position that will afford them the most comfort. A seat directly above a wheel arch will generally be more susceptible to vibrations. Likewise, a seat on the offside of the vehicle is likely to be more comfortable due to most road defects, drain covers for example, being nearest to the kerb.

If seats in the vehicle are of different heights, try to ensure that patients can reach the floor with their feet, enabling them to gain better stability when the vehicle is cornering, and point out any handrails that may be available to them.

Patients on a stretcher can feel vulnerable and insecure, especially as they are rear-facing. Ensure that they are securely fastened in with the securing belts/harnesses provided and, if their condition permits, that they are sitting up on the stretcher.

Knowledge recap questions

1. Describe three specialist skills that emergency response drivers should possess.

2. How frequently should drivers perform dynamic risk assessments?

3. Describe two types of operational stress that drivers may encounter while carrying out their day-to-day duties.

4. Describe two tactics that can be used by drivers to deal with the effects of stress.

5. Why must the comfort of patients be taken into consideration when formulating driving plans?

6. How can different seating positions within an ambulance affect passenger comfort?

4 Vehicle Daily Inspections and Pre-Driving Checks

Carrying out simple, comprehensive checks on the vehicles that you drive is key to ensuring the roadworthiness of those vehicles and the safety of the crew and patients that they carry.

While individual Trusts may have set inspection procedures that you must follow, this chapter outlines what should be checked, how frequently it should be done, and the reasons why these checks are carried out.

Learning outcomes

By the end of this chapter you should:

▲ Identify how to carry out a vehicle daily inspection (VDI) and describe why it is important and necessary.

▲ Perform the seven stages of a VDI.

▲ Identify how to carry out a pre-driving check (PDC) and describe why it is important and necessary.

▲ Perform the ten stages of a PDC.

Vehicle daily inspection

A VDI should be conducted at the start of each shift or every time a different vehicle is driven. Once practised it should take no more than ten minutes.

Any defects found during the VDI should be noted and reported via the Trust's reporting procedure in order for remedial action to be undertaken. A vehicle should not be driven with a dangerous or illegal defect.

Item to check	What to do	Why
1. Visual examination of the exterior	As you approach the vehicle check that it sits correctly on the ground and isn't leaning to one side or to the front/back. Look under the vehicle for any obvious fluid leaks. While conducting the other checks described below, check for damage to the bodywork.	If the vehicle is leaning to one side or to the front/back, this could indicate a problem with the suspension. Signs of fluid on the floor underneath the vehicle could indicate a water or oil leak requiring further examination. Damage to bodywork can be dangerous to other road users, particularly if there are sharp edges left after collision damage. All body panels, lights and bumpers should be securely attached to ensure they don't fall off when the vehicle is moving.

Item to check	What to do	Why
2. Wheels and tyres	Make sure that each wheel has all wheel nuts present and that they are secure. If the vehicle is fitted with telltale markers, ensure they all point in the correct direction.

Check that the wheel rims are in good condition and free from cracks to the metalwork.

Check tyres for correct and legal tread depth (1.6mm across the centre three-quarters of the tyre*), correct pressure and overall condition.

*Most Trusts replace tyres at 3mm. | Due to the arduous working conditions an ambulance is subject to, wheel damage is a possibility and so should be checked for.

When a tyre is replaced, a missing or incorrectly tightened wheel nut could cause the wheel to work free, causing a collision. It is also important to check the wheel rims for security and damage.

Tyres are vitally important to the correct handling, stopping and accelerating characteristics of the vehicle – an unidentified fault in tread depth, pressure or damage could have serious consequences. |

Item to check	What to do	Why
3. Under-bonnet checks	With the engine cold (or stopped for at least ten minutes) and the vehicle parked on a level surface, check that the oil, coolant, brake and hydraulic fluid levels are all between the minimum and maximum. Ideally they should be above half. Check that the windscreen washer fluid is topped up.	Inaccurate results may be found if these checks are completed when the engine is warm or on a slope. A lack of oil or coolant could result in serious engine damage or failure. A lack of brake or hydraulic fluid could mean that the brakes or power steering don't work effectively. Having the washer bottle topped up will ensure that you can clean the windscreen as required.
4. Lights	Ensure that all lights function to include: ● Sidelights, headlights, tail lights, fog lights ● High beam ● Brake lights ● Indicators and hazard warning lights ● Daytime running lights ● Emergency warning lights (where fitted) ● Interior and map-reading lights.	In most cases it is a legal requirement for the lights to be fully functioning. It is also important as they enable you to see, be seen and give indication to others of your intentions.

Item to check	What to do	Why
5. Windscreen, windows and mirrors, and wipers	Ensure that the windscreen is free from cracks and chips, and is clean and clear. Ensure that all other windows and mirrors are free from cracks and chips, and are clean and clear. Ensure that the windscreen wipers function correctly and that the washer system, where fitted, works. (Ensure windscreen is wet.) Check the tax disc is in date and appropriate while inspecting the windscreen. (Paper tax disks will no longer be issued from 1st October 2014.)	It is vitally important that you can see clearly out of all windows. When undertaking emergency driving at night or in poor weather conditions an unclean windscreen can cause the driver significant problems with visibility, meaning a reduction in progress. Checking for cracks and chips is important as they may make the vehicle un-roadworthy and require a replacement to be fitted.
6. Horn	Check that the horn and sirens, where fitted, work correctly.	It is important to check that the sirens and horn work before they are required.

Item to check	What to do	Why
7. Ambulance equipment	Check the presence, security and function of any safety or ambulance-specific equipment.	This is your opportunity to check things such as the first aid kit, fire extinguisher and medical equipment, as fitted to the grade of vehicle you are driving.

Pre-driving check (PDC)

The completion of a PDC, or cockpit check/drill, will ensure that you are familiar with the location of all of the vehicle controls and can operate them all effectively. It will also help to ensure the safety and comfort of the crew and passengers.

A PDC should be completed the first time that an unfamiliar vehicle is driven, or at the start of your shift. It need not be completed in full every time you enter the vehicle, providing no one else has driven the vehicle in the interim.

When preparing to drive a vehicle that you have previously driven that day/night, and providing that no one else has driven it since, only points 1, 5 and 9 need to be completed.

There will be some variation on the list provided in the table below depending upon the vehicle but, in general, all items should be checked or adjusted.

Item to check	What to do	Why
1. Handbrake and neutral gear	Upon entering the vehicle ensure that the handbrake is applied and the gear lever is in neutral (or 'park' in an automatic).	It is important to ensure that the vehicle is secure. The additional weight of a person entering the vehicle could cause it to move, especially if it is parked on a hill. Checking for neutral will ensure that if the vehicle is started inadvertently it won't lurch forwards.

Item to check	What to do	Why
2. Seat position and steering wheel	Adjust your seat so that you are comfortable and can reach the controls easily. Your seating position should also enable you to have a good all-round view. **Seat height:** ● Adjust this so that you can see out of the front and side windows clearly. **Seat base:** ● Adjust this so that the clutch (or brake in an automatic vehicle) can be fully depressed and you have a slight bend at the knee. **Seat back:** ● Adjust this in conjunction with the steering wheel height/rake adjustment. You should have a slight bend in your elbows with your hands in the 'ten to two' position on the steering wheel.	It is important that your seat is correctly adjusted so that you are able to use the controls effectively. For example, you must be able to fully depress the clutch and have unhindered rotation of the steering wheel with your hands. A correctly adjusted seat position is also important for protection in the event of a collision. For example, a correctly adjusted head restraint can help to reduce, or even eliminate, whiplash injuries. Finally, a comfortable seating position will reduce driver fatigue and enable you to concentrate fully on the task in hand.

Item to check	What to do	Why
2. Seat position and steering wheel *continued*	**Head restraint:** • Adjust this so that the top of the head restraint is in line with your eye line. **Lumbar support:** • Adjust this so that you are comfortable. Ensure that all controls for seat adjustment are firmly in position and that the seat won't move when you move off or brake heavily.	
3. Mirrors	**Internal rear-view mirror:** • Hold the outside rim of the mirror with your left hand and adjust it so that the top edge is aligned with the top edge of the rear window. You should be able to frame the rear window left to right – if you can't, go for a right bias.	Having a good view all around your vehicle is essential for safe driving. Correct mirror adjustment will also enable you to find reference points when reversing, which will make it safer and more convenient for you when manoeuvring.

Item to check	What to do	Why
3. Mirrors *continued*	• If your vehicle has a mirror provided for you to observe the rear saloon (such as in an ambulance) ensure that this is adjusted for maximum vision. **Exterior mirrors:** • Adjust these so that you can see the side of the vehicle in one third and the road in the other two-thirds. • They should be adjusted to minimise any blind spots and should be aligned so that you can see the top of the rear wheel arch. • If the mirrors are electronically adjusted you may need to turn the ignition on, remembering to turn it off again once the mirrors have been suitably aligned.	You should be aware of your vehicle's blind spots – the areas that cannot be seen in your mirrors or when looking forwards.

Item to check	What to do	Why
3. Mirrors *continued*	Note whether the vehicle is fitted with wide-angle mirrors or other blind-spot detection systems and ensure that you are familiar with their operation.	
4. Gearbox familiarisation and confirmation of neutral	**Manual vehicle:** • Take hold of the gear lever in your left hand. Put it into neutral and move it from side to side once to note the large lateral movement. Then engage a forward gear, normally first. Note the small lateral movement. Now move the gear lever back to neutral and ensure that it rests normally between third and fourth gear. • Ensure that you know where reverse gear is and how to select it.	It is important to know the type of gearbox fitted to the vehicle, the number of gears and the location of reverse, as there may be different types within your ambulance service. Engaging first gear will help you to identify the condition of the gearbox and allow for confirmation of neutral. It is important to ensure that the vehicle is in neutral (or 'park' for automatics) before starting the engine, otherwise it could lurch forwards.

Item to check	What to do	Why
4. Gearbox familiarisation and confirmation of neutral *continued*	Automatic vehicle: ● Take hold of the gear selector with your left hand. Ensure that it is in 'P' or 'park' mode. ● Note the gear selector options and the type of gearbox fitted to the vehicle.	
5. Starting the vehicle	Fully depress the clutch pedal (or the brake in an automatic vehicle). With the key inserted, turn the ignition on so that the dashboard illuminates and the steering lock is released. Note the self-check function of the vehicle diagnostics, ensuring that all lights that should go out do so (model dependent). Ensure that all auxiliary devices, such as the ventilation controls, radio and ambulance equipment, are switched to the 'off' position.	When starting the engine it is important to ensure safety. By depressing the clutch (or the brake in an automatic) you are disengaging the engine from the drive train – doing so ensures that the vehicle will remain stationary when started if the vehicle is in a false neutral or the gear linkage is broken. By applying light downward pressure to the steering wheel when you start the engine you should get feedback from the steering system indicating that the power steering pump is functioning.

Item to check	What to do	Why
5. Starting the vehicle *continued*	Do not apply pressure to the accelerator as the engine management system will apply the correct degree of fuel to start the vehicle. Apply the footbrake and hold the steering wheel firmly with one hand applying slight pressure downwards. Start the engine with the other hand, either by pressing the start button or turning the key. Ensure that all of the dashboard warning lights have extinguished with the exception of the handbrake warning light. Gently release the clutch pedal but continue to keep the brake pedal depressed. Ensure that all gauges are working and that there is sufficient fuel for your journey.	Depressing the clutch and ensuring that all auxiliary equipment is turned off before starting the engine will remove any unnecessary electrical or mechanical load on the vehicle, making it easier to start, particularly in cold weather. It is also important to check that all lights are extinguished as any lights that remain on might indicate a problem with the vehicle's engine or electrical systems. If any lights do remain on you should consult the vehicle's handbook.

Item to check	What to do	Why
6. Static brake test	Depress the brake pedal fully three times with your right foot, keeping it engaged on the last press. Once the pedal is fully depressed there should be no movement in the brake pedal – the pedal should feel firm underfoot. Maintain pressure on the brake pedal while you conduct item 7.	It is important to check for problems with the hydraulic braking circuit. If the pedal is not firm underfoot, this may indicate a problem.
7. Handbrake test	With the footbrake fully applied, release the handbrake with your left hand by applying a slight upward lift and depressing the pawl release button with your thumb. Allow the handbrake to travel to the fully 'off' position and then reapply it, again depressing the pawl release button. Note the normal position for the handbrake when in the 'on' position.	You now know that the handbrake can be released and, when you reapply it, you know the position at which the vehicle will be secured. If you detected any movement in the footbrake pedal or a change in pressure, this might indicate a problem with the braking system.

Item to check	What to do	Why
7. Handbrake test *continued*	In a vehicle with an electrically operated handbrake, ensure you know how to operate it – disengage and reapply it to ensure its function.	
8. Auxiliary controls	Working from left to right, ensure that you are familiar with all controls fitted to the vehicle. Key areas to check include: ● Ventilation controls, air conditioning, heating ● Indicators, lights, hazard lights, fog lights ● Windscreen wipers and washers ● Interior lights, map-reading lights ● Storage compartments, sun visors ● Emergency warning lights, sirens, horn ● Communication equipment, data head	It is vital that you know how to operate every control in your vehicle. When responding to an emergency your mind must be on the task of driving; you should not have to divert attention to finding an auxiliary control such as the ventilation system – these should fall to hand. It is highly likely that you will drive many different vehicles, often in a single day, with different set-ups – you must be familiar with their controls before you start your journey.

Item to check	What to do	Why
8. Auxiliary controls *continued*	• Mobile phone holders, Bluetooth connection • Entertainment radio, satellite navigation. Ensure that there is nothing likely to hinder your use of the controls, such as kit bags on the floor, and that everything is stowed safely away. Check the condition of the floor covering and that there is nothing likely to roll under the pedals.	
9. Seat belt and doors	Take hold of the seat belt buckle with your left hand. Fully withdraw the webbing, paying attention to any tears, rips or frayed areas. Insert the buckle into the locking mechanism and release to ensure that the locking mechanism is functioning. Now reinsert the buckle to secure the seat belt.	A correctly adjusted seat belt helps to reduce or avoid injury should the vehicle be involved in a collision. For the seat belt pre-tensioners and airbags to work correctly, the occupant must be in the correct position – the seat belt ensures that this is the case.

Item to check	What to do	Why
9. **Seat belt and doors** *continued*	Adjust the seat belt so that the lap belt sits across your abdomen and the upper restraint sits across your sternum. The seat belt should be close fitting. If available, adjust the seat belt height setting so that it is 25mm above your right shoulder.	Vehicles may suffer from premature seat belt wear because of the high number of short journeys they undertake and because of the equipment clinicians often carry on their belts.
10. **Mobile brake test**	Check that all of the doors are shut. Before moving on to the road network, conduct a mobile brake test: • Check your mirrors and accelerate to around 20mph. • Checking your mirrors again and, warning your passengers, apply the brakes in a firm (but not emergency) manner. • Check that the vehicle pulls up in the expected distance and that it stops in a straight line.	A mobile brake test will confirm that the brakes are working effectively.

Item to check	What to do	Why
10. Mobile brake test *continued*	Be aware of increased stopping distances in poor weather and ensure that there is suitable room to conduct this manoeuvre in all circumstances. If there is not the room to conduct this test in an off-road environment, consider braking early and gently for the first hazard or junction on your journey.	

Knowledge recap questions

1. How frequently should a vehicle daily inspection be carried out?

2. What should you do if you find a defect during a vehicle daily inspection?

3. Why should vehicles be parked on a level surface when carrying out checks of fluids under the bonnet?

4. How frequently should a PDC be carried out?

5. State two reasons why a correctly adjusted seat position is important.

6. What is a blind spot?

7. Why should you fully depress the clutch pedal when starting a manual transmission vehicle?

5 Automatic Gearboxes

Many ambulance vehicles are fitted with an automatic transmission; these replace the need for a conventional clutch and gearbox so the driver no longer has to shift gears manually. It is important that adequate training is received in their use in order to drive the vehicles correctly and safely.

As automatic gearboxes are becoming more common it is essential that drivers know how to make the best use of them. This chapter outlines the general principles of automatic gearboxes – understanding them will enable drivers to make the correct decisions based on accurate driving plans with due consideration to the presence of various hazards and the performance of the vehicle.

Learning outcomes

By the end of this chapter you should:

▲ Understand the functionality of selector options.

▲ Know the principles of how and when to manually lock down the gears.

▲ Recognise the important characteristics of automatic gearboxes.

▲ Know the difference between manual and automatic transmissions with regards to 'creep', 'run on' and 'kick down'.

▲ Understand how to get the most out of an automatic transmission when driving an emergency response vehicle.

Selector options

The selector control may be located on the dashboard, floor or steering column, an example of which can be seen in Figure 5.1. Some vehicles have paddles or push-button mechanisms. An illuminated indicator panel (usually mounted on the dashboard) provides visual confirmation of the position currently selected.

As discussed, there are variations to the location of controls in automatic vehicles but the function principles remain the same.

The basic selector positions are:

- **P (PARK)** – this should be selected when the vehicle is parked, before the engine is switched off. A check should be made that the selector is in this position before attempting to start the engine. To further ensure safety, the footbrake should be depressed while starting the engine. **Never move the lever to the 'P' position while the vehicle is in motion.**

- **R (REVERSE)** – this is usually located next to 'park' in the selector mechanism sequence. The footbrake must always be depressed when moving the selector from 'P' to 'R', or when moving from 'P' through 'R' to get to another selector option. **The vehicle will begin to move backwards the instant the selector is moved into 'R', unless the brakes are applied.**

- **N (NEUTRAL)** – no power is transmitted from the engine to the drive wheels when in 'neutral'. It should be selected when the vehicle needs to be towed after a breakdown or accident. It should not be selected when making temporary stops in traffic.

- **D (DRIVE)** – this is the regular operational mode when driving an automatic under normal driving conditions. It allows the transmission to make automatic adjustments according to your speed, engine loading and accelerator position. As the accelerator is depressed, and the vehicle gathers speed, sensors detect the optimum time to change up to the next highest gear. The change is made automatically, without the intervention of the driver. Changes can be detected by watching the rev counter and listening for changes in the engine note. Harsh acceleration can result in jerky changes, while smooth and gradual increases in speed may make changes imperceptible to patients and other passengers.

Not remaining neutral

Remember that there is no need to move the gear lever into 'neutral' when stationary in traffic, even for many minutes. No wear is taking place; in fact, more wear will take place if you put it into 'neutral' then back into 'drive' when you are ready to move off. Most gearboxes will automatically select first gear when your vehicle stops in anticipation of your next movement.

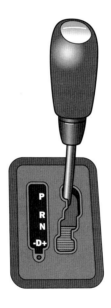

Figure 5.1   An example of the four positions of the selector lever:

P – Park: prevents the vehicle from rolling away when stopped

R – Reverse: only engage reverse gear when the vehicle is stationary

N – Neutral: no power is transmitted from the engine to the drive wheels

D – Drive: automatic drive using all forward gears and a configuration of 1, 2, 3 and 4 for manual selection, or a plus or minus sign for upward or downward manual changes, allowing the vehicle to be driven like a clutchless manual vehicle.

Safety warning

It is vitally important to remember that automatics do not have a clutch pedal. Depressing the footbrake with the left foot, in the mistaken belief that this is the clutch, can have disastrous consequences – particularly if the vehicle is being driven at speed and being followed too closely by another road user.

Automatics should always be left in 'park' ('P') when not being driven. When carrying out a PDC, 'selector in P' should be substituted for 'gear lever in neutral'.

Manual gear select

In many instances the gear selector can remain in 'D' but there are clearly occasions when the manual selection of gears is required to maximise flexibility, stability and control of the vehicle. This feature essentially enables an automatic vehicle to be driven like a clutchless manual vehicle. The vehicle's manual will describe how to manually change down and limit the range of gear ratios.

This is an effective means of controlling an automatic gearbox while descending steep gradients or overtaking. The number of lock down options varies and depends on whether the vehicle being driven has four, five or six gears. The number of lock down options will always be less than the total number of gears present: a five-speed gearbox will have four lock down options while a vehicle with four gears will have three lock down choices.

- **Lock down 1** – This is used on very steep downhill gradients to utilise engine compression to help control speed and lessen the load on the brakes. The vehicle should be brought to a halt at the top of the slope before selecting lock down 1.

  In lock down 1 the vehicle is locked in first gear and will not change up to any other gear. The selector should be moved back to 'drive' when the descent has been completed.

- **Lock down 2** – This is used to control speed on descents in the same way as lock down 1. As the gear is higher, there is less engine compression. This option is suitable for fairly steep downhill gradients – the selector will not change up to third or any higher gear.

- **Lock down 3** – This is used for overtaking in a vehicle fitted with four gears. It can also be used for controlling speed on moderate downhill gradients in a vehicle fitted with five or more gears. Overtaking in an automatic can be more hazardous than when driving a vehicle fitted with manual transmission. This is because as speed is increased to complete the manoeuvre, the automatic gearbox is predisposed to change up to the next highest gear, which can result in a potentially disastrous loss of power at a critical point in the overtake. Using a lock down option before beginning to overtake eliminates this possibility. The selector should be moved back to 'drive' when the manoeuvre has been completed safely.

- **Lock down 4/5** – This is used for overtaking, as described above, in vehicles fitted with five or six gears.

You might choose to lock down a lower gear in a built-up area, where there are a number of hazards, to improve control through the accelerator. However, the gear you select should always be appropriate for your circumstances. In a five-speed automatic box, third gear may be most suitable for urban driving while fourth may be a better and more flexible choice for rural roads.

It is essential to remember to move the selector back to 'drive' when the need to utilise lock down has passed. Driving the vehicle for a prolonged period in a lock down option can overheat the automatic transmission fluid and cause damage to the transmission system.

Moving the selector is best done when not accelerating. Care must be taken to ensure that the selector is moved the correct number of steps to reach the desired position. The gear selected must be appropriate for the speed that you are travelling at – most modern systems will override your lever selection if the engine revs or speed are too high.

Practice is essential to facilitate accuracy when attention cannot be diverted from the road ahead to check the indicator panel.

> ### REMEMBER!
> **With both automatic and manual gearboxes, you must be travelling at the correct speed for the gear that you want to select manually. Secondary braking should be avoided.**

Important characteristics of automatic gearboxes

Creep

If any selector position other than 'P' or 'N' is selected, and the footbrake or handbrake are not applied, then the vehicle will tend to creep forward or backward at low speed, even when pressure is not applied to the accelerator pedal.

The rate of creep varies in response to the force of gravity. Consequently, creep will be greater on a downhill slope than an uphill slope. Creep can, and must, be controlled by using the footbrake. It is particularly useful when manoeuvring at low speeds or when negotiating obstacles such as ramps and speed bumps.

Run on

Deceleration in a vehicle fitted with manual transmission is relatively straightforward – releasing pressure on the accelerator pedal slows the engine and deceleration is achieved by means of engine compression. This is especially effective in lower gears. This is not the case in an automatic when driving an automatic with the selector set in the 'D' position, however. Releasing pressure on the accelerator will not result in a change down to a lower gear, nor is engine compression apparent.

This is referred to as 'run on' and provides a driving sensation similar to 'coasting'. If the vehicle is travelling uphill, gravity will slow it down. If the vehicle is travelling downhill, however, the combined effects of run on and gravity will result in a progressive increase in speed. Steep downward slopes can produce an alarming sensation of losing control as gravity takes over and vehicle speed rises sharply.

The timely and judicious use of lock down (see above) will effectively prevent this potentially dangerous circumstance. When driving on level stretches of road, early relaxation of pressure on the accelerator will facilitate more efficient acceleration sense.

Kick down

This is a useful safety feature that should only be used at times of actual or potential danger. It provides short-term bursts of maximum acceleration, to escape from hazardous circumstances, without the need to move the selector lever.

'Kick' the accelerator pedal down rapidly and forcefully to the furthest limit of its travel. After a very brief interval the transmission will change down to the next lowest gear and rapid acceleration will ensue. Holding the pedal down may result in a further subsequent change down and yet more acceleration. You then have a mechanism to escape from danger by using maximum acceleration when this is appropriate. Relaxing pressure on the accelerator results in loss of acceleration and a change back up to a higher gear.

Key terms

Creep – the tendency of an automatic vehicle to creep forwards or backwards at low speed, even when pressure is not applied to the accelerator.

Run on – the tendency of an automatic vehicle not to reduce speed when pressure is no longer applied to the accelerator; the vehicle may even gain speed if travelling downhill.

Kick down – a feature of automatic vehicles that allows you to suddenly accelerate quickly, overriding the automatic selection of gears.

Care must be taken when using kick down. Plan and look well ahead to ensure that the vehicle is not powered out of one dangerous situation and into another.

Automatic vehicles and their application in emergency response driving

Although some police forces advocate a more direct manual use of automatic boxes, particularly in response situations, the manual override facility should not be used excessively. If you do not require a greater degree of flexibility or maximum performance from the vehicle, you should consider carefully whether it is really necessary.

While it is impossible to provide gear selection guidance for all eventualities, the following advice is intended to provide some general guidance in some common sets of circumstances:

- **Control over speed:** when you need more control over acceleration – for example in response to a particular hazard, when overtaking or approaching an area of uncertainty – manually selecting a particular gear will prevent the gearbox from changing up automatically, providing more flexibility to control speed. Once need for this flexibility has passed, however, the 'D' option should be reconsidered.

- **Stopping:** apply the footbrake before moving the gear lever when the vehicle is stationary. Set the handbrake (for temporary stops longer than ten seconds) as many automatic vehicles will creep and some have a tendency to lurch. Leave the selector in 'D' when stopped in traffic, at junctions and at traffic lights. There is no need to move into neutral.

- **At roundabouts:** engage the appropriate gear in manual mode on the approach to the hazard to provide greater vehicle stability.

- **On bends:** gentle bends can normally be negotiated in 'D'. For a series of bends, however, manually select a suitable gear before the first bend; on exiting that bend, when the accelerator is eased in preparation for the next bend, the vehicle will not automatically change up. This provides the benefit of engine braking, which gives better control.

- **Overtaking:** when overtaking you can choose to either manually select a lower gear or use the 'kick down' function. If you need to accelerate then decelerate rapidly to fit into a gap, manually selecting a lower gear before the start of the manoeuvre may be beneficial.

- **Steep hills:** when descending steep hills in 'D', automatic vehicles have a tendency to change into a higher gear, which can necessitate the need for excessive braking. This can induce 'brake fade' – a reduction in stopping power after sustained or repeated braking. This can be overcome by manually locking down to a low ratio gear, which will then provide compression braking to enhance vehicle braking. Similarly, when ascending steep hills, locking a ratio manually can provide better control.

- Never select 'P' while the vehicle is in motion. It will cause major damage or an accident by locking the transmission.

- Only engage reverse gear when the vehicle is stationary, otherwise the transmission could be damaged.

- Ensure that the footbrake is on before engaging either 'D' or 'R' from stationary.

- Do not engage 'D' or 'R' with a high-revving engine.

- Check that you do not knock the gear lever accidentally as this could change the gear out of 'D' to fourth.

Manually selecting a gear can be useful in circumstances when the gearbox is continually changing up and down between two gears; this can also reduce wear on the gearbox.

It is not always necessary to manually select a lower gear for a hazard as you might do when driving a manual vehicle. Modern automatic gearboxes are designed to select the correct ratio for the speed and throttle setting.

Key term

Brake fade – a reduction in stopping power after sustained or repeated braking.

However, manual selection should be considered if this would offer better stability for the vehicle in respect of the circumstances encountered at the time.

It is not possible to determine all the occasions when 'D' compared to manual gears should be selected. Drivers must execute accurate judgement and use of driving plans to judge which is most appropriate. Avoid making unnecessary or excessive use of the manual hold position – you should return to 'D' when the need has passed.

Automatics can make driving appear easier by removing the need to make recurring changes of gear while concentrating on maintaining smooth clutch control. Diligent application of the above principles will ensure that you get the best from your vehicle while maintaining full control without compromising safety margins.

Knowledge recap questions

1. Name the four basic gear selector positions in an automatic vehicle.

2. What would happen if the gear lever was moved into the 'P' (park) position while the vehicle was in motion?

3. In what circumstances would you select the 'N' (neutral) position?

4. Why should you always consider moving the gear selector back to 'D' (drive) after a period of lock down?

5. What is 'creep' and how can it be avoided?

6. Releasing pressure on the accelerator of a manual vehicle usually results in the vehicle slowing down. Why is this not always the case for automatic vehicles?

7. In what circumstances might you utilise an automatic vehicle's 'kick down' function?

6 Vehicle Operating and Safety Systems

The NHS ambulance service has evolved considerably over the years, from operating a fleet of vehicles specifically designed for the purpose of conveying patients to a range of bespoke vehicles including response cars, resilience vehicles, motorcycles and covert vehicles among many others.

In this chapter we consider some of the vehicle operating systems and safety features that you are likely to encounter when driving ambulance vehicles. These include the key fob, braking and stability systems, electrical control systems, Emergency Warning Equipment controls and dashboard warning lights.

Learning outcomes

By the end of this chapter you should:

▲ Be able to identify the various types of braking and brake assist systems.

▲ Recognise the various dashboard warning lamps that indicate brake system malfunctions.

▲ Understand the purpose of retarder systems.

▲ Understand the various vehicle stability and traction control features.

▲ Know how to operate the run lock system.

▲ Demonstrate how to connect electrical charge support systems to the vehicle and isolate the batteries.

▲ Correctly operate all emergency lighting controls.

▲ Identify the various electrical emergency warning malfunction lights and take the appropriate action.

The key fob

Figure 6.1 illustrates an example of a standard ambulance key fob.

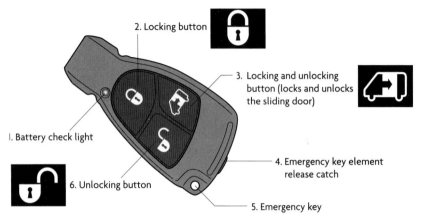

2. Locking button

3. Locking and unlocking button (locks and unlocks the sliding door)

I. Battery check light

6. Unlocking button

4. Emergency key element release catch

5. Emergency key

Figure 6.1 Key fob.

At the top edge of the fob is a slide button; when moved it releases the key within the fob. This key opens the driver door should the fob fail to operate due to battery malfunction or damage.

Care should be given not to leave the key fob in the vehicle; the vehicle may automatically lock if all the doors are closed.

Brake systems

Most modern ambulance vehicles offer a number of safety systems to assist with vehicle braking. Figure 6.2 provides an example of typical dashboard warning lights that identify some of these systems. Note that this is intended to provide an example and that there are other similar systems in operation.

Brake assist system

The brake assist system (BAS) is designed to operate during emergency braking situations. When the brake pedal is depressed quickly the BAS automatically increases the brake pressure, reducing the stopping distance.

If the BAS malfunctions or fails, the vehicle will still have its full brake effect but the stopping distance may increase.

Antilock brake system

When the antilock brake system (ABS) is activated this enables the driver to steer and brake without the wheels locking during harsh braking; a pulsating of the brake pedal will be experienced. ABS is designed to be the technical equivalent to 'cadence braking'.

Electronic brakeforce distribution

Electronic brakeforce distribution (EBD) monitors and controls the brake pressure placed upon the wheels to improve vehicle handling while braking.

 ESP malfunction

 ASR or BAS malfunction

 Brake fluid level low or EBD malfunction

 ABS malfunction

 Brake pads/linings worn

Figure 6.2   Dashboard warning signals.

Retarders

Retarders – sometimes called exhaust brakes – are often fitted to large vehicles; they assist the braking systems by helping to slow the vehicle down at all road speeds while ensuring a smooth ride. The system is often fully automatic and the control system is normally activated by the action of the driver depressing the brake pedal and requires no additional driver operations and no special training other than an awareness of it to enhance understanding of this additional safety system.

The standstill system automatically detects when the vehicle is moving, preparing the retarder system for use.

The retarder system reaction time is virtually instantaneous. This makes for optimum compatibility with ABS. Application of the footbrake operates the circuits in the control box, which close, and energises the retarder, which applies the 'friction-free' braking torque to the rear wheels, slowing the vehicle down. In most vehicles there is a red 'R' switch which will illuminate during this function; it is normally situated close to the instrument panel (see Figure 6.3).

You should ensure that you know what type of system is fitted to your vehicle and follow any manufacturer-specific instructions.

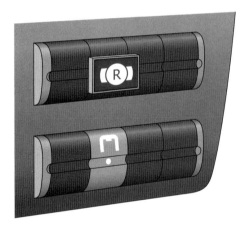

Figure 6.3 The red 'R' switch.

Retarder systems have, in some instances, been shown to automatically absorb over 80% of braking applications. This helps in keeping brake temperatures low. High brake temperatures lead to brake wear, maintenance costs and increased vehicle downtime.

Retarder systems can also help reduce overall stopping distances, provided that tyre adhesion is maintained, giving obvious benefits to the crew, medical staff, patients and other road users. In tests carried out under relatively heavy service braking levels of 50%, at a speed of just 30mph, the retarder can reduce the total stopping distance by 3m.

The system slows the vehicle via the rear axle and, when braking, contributes to keeping the vehicle level, eliminating most of the front-end 'dipping'. This provides a considerable improvement in vehicle stability when braking, both in a straight line and when cornering, with reduced 'roll' of the vehicle and a greater sense of confidence in the overall handling.

Traction control systems

Most modern vehicles are equipped with various stability systems that are designed to assist with maximising traction while the vehicle is in motion.

Acceleration skid control

Acceleration skid control (ASR) is designed to improve vehicle traction, which means that the power from the tyres is transferred to the road surface for a set period. This results in improved stability of the vehicle. ASR also assists when moving off and accelerating, especially on smooth or slippery surfaces. ASR works by applying brake effect to individual drive wheels and reducing the engine torque to prevent the drive wheels from spinning.

A warning light in the instrument cluster flashes when ASR is active. As ASR is a safety feature fitted to the vehicle, it must not be deactivated.

Electronic stability programme

The electronic stability programme (ESP) is another vehicle safety system that works by monitoring vehicle stability. It is able to predict when the vehicle may under- or oversteer, which could result in the vehicle skidding. It works by recovering vehicle stability by braking individual wheels and reducing power output from the engine.

The system is valuable when driving on wet or slippery road surfaces where tyre grip is reduced. Similar to an ASR system, a warning light flashes when the system is active. It is important to understand that this system can't remove the risk of a collision – if the vehicle speed is excessive or inappropriate for the road conditions, ESP will not work. It is not possible to override the laws of physics!

Run lock systems

Emergency vehicles are often equipped with a run lock system, which allows the driver to remove the ignition key for security reasons while the engine continues to operate to maintain electrical charge. This is of particular importance in modern-day ambulance vehicles due to the extensive range of electrical equipment fitted, such as data systems, telecommunications, medical devices, heating and emergency warning lights.

In the event of an attempted theft of the vehicle, the engine would cut out if the vehicle was to be driven away.

You should follow your service's guidelines when using these systems to ensure compliance with policy and law.

Electrical and emergency lighting control systems

Due to the volume and variety of electrical equipment fitted to modern emergency ambulance vehicles and the subsequent power demand, especially while stationary, many vehicles are fitted with a number of batteries.

- **Emergency start button** – the emergency start button can be utilised if a battery drain is affecting engine ignition; power is sourced from an auxiliary battery that should be sufficient to start the vehicle.

- **Electrical umbilical leads** – while stationary and parked for prolonged periods, such as at ambulance stations, emergency vehicles should be connected to umbilical electrical charge leads where available. They ensure the batteries receive constant charge. Although the lead system is designed to automatically disconnect when the engine starts, confirmation of this must be established as part of the moving-off procedure.

- **Isolators** – most vehicles will also be equipped with isolation switches which can be used for emergency isolation if required or to preserve battery power when vehicles are parked for extensive periods.

Emergency lighting controls

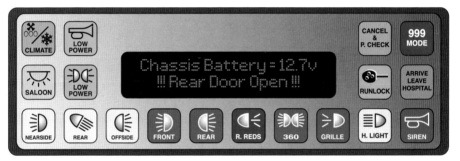

Figure 6.4   Lighting controls.

Cancel and pre-check

This is a special feature button that can only be activated when the ignition and handbrake are both on.

When pressed and held for five seconds it activates every function that can be visually inspected, individually and sequentially in a predetermined order.

Arrive/leave hospital mode

If the ignition is on, when this mode is selected the ignition security feature is the first function to be activated, allowing you to remove the ignition key and leave the engine running securely. Depending on the specification, the engine's speed may increase from idle. This will obviously not operate if the vehicle is in gear (or 'D' selected in an automatic).

If the handbrake is released the engine will stall.

Siren activation

When the siren is activated; the sound/tone can normally be changed by pressing the vehicle horn or, on older models, by pressing the button where the clutch pedal would normally be on a manual vehicle.

Risk of collisions

To reduce the risk of collisions, remember that if any of the icons below light up while on a journey, there may be a malfunction in the EBD. You should drive with particular care and ensure that the fault is investigated as soon as possible.

Figure 6.5   Warning lights.

If any of these warning lights in the instrument cluster flash, you should proceed as follows:

● Do not deactivate ASR under any circumstances

● Depress the accelerator pedal only as far as necessary when pulling away

● Adapt your driving style to suit the road and weather conditions, otherwise the vehicle could start to skid.

If the ESP indicator icon is constantly lit when the engine is running, there is a malfunction, which may mean that engine power output is reduced. The fault needs to be investigated as soon as possible.

> **REMEMBER!**
> **If ASR is deactivated there is an increased risk that the brake system of the vehicle could overheat and could be damaged, compromising vehicle safety.**

Knowledge recap questions

1. Name three features that are normally found in emergency response vehicles to assist the braking system.

2. Describe what happens if the brake assist system (BAS) malfunctions.

3. Describe how retarder systems work.

4. Why should high brake temperatures be avoided?

5. Describe how acceleration skid control (ASR) works and why it must not be deactivated under any circumstances.

6. What is the purpose of a run lock system?

7. Why should emergency vehicles be connected to umbilical electrical charge leads when stationary or parked for prolonged periods at an ambulance station?

7 Audible and Visual Warnings

The presence of an emergency vehicle often influences the behaviour of other road users and pedestrians and, for these reasons, emergency ambulances are fitted with visual and/or audible warnings to alert road users to your presence or approach.

In this chapter we consider the active and passive visual warnings that are incorporated into ambulances, as well as their audible warnings, and the impact that they can have on other road users.

Learning outcomes

By the end of this chapter you should:

▲ Understand the purpose and use of passive visual warnings.

▲ Understand the purpose and use of active visual warnings.

▲ Understand the purpose and use of audible warnings.

▲ Recognise the benefit of alternating siren tones.

▲ Know the risks associated with travelling in convoy in relation to siren use.

▲ Recognise when the use of Emergency Warning Equipment is permitted.

▲ Recognise when Emergency Warning Equipment must not be used and when the deactivation of sirens should be considered.

Appearance and markings

Visual warnings on an ambulance can be of two types – passive or active.

Passive visual warnings

Passive visual warnings are incorporated into the design of the vehicle and usually involve high-contrast patterns. The designs may be painted on to older ambulances, but modern ambulances generally have retro-reflective designs that reflect light from car headlights. Popular patterns include:

- 'Checkerboard' or 'Battenberg' – alternate coloured squares

- Chevrons or arrowheads

- Stripes along the side.

In addition to this, many emergency service vehicles are painted a bright (sometimes fluorescent) yellow or orange for maximum visual impact.

Another passive visual warning is the word 'ambulance' spelled out in reverse on the front of the vehicle. This enables drivers in front of the approaching ambulance to identify it in their rear-view mirrors more easily.

It is important to remember that the bright yellow colouring and markings on ambulances may be suddenly noticed by traffic ahead of you. This can sometimes be after a prolonged period of non-observance, resulting in sudden or unexpected vehicle movement or braking without warning. It is therefore important that adequate following distances are maintained.

Similarly, other services have adopted the 'checkerboard' or 'Battenberg' designs, such as the police with blue and yellow, the fire service with red and yellow, and the Highways Agency with black and yellow.

Active visual warnings

Flashing coloured lights – known as 'beacons' or 'light bars' – are the most obvious visual feature fitted to emergency ambulance vehicles. Their purpose is to attract the attention of other road users and to warn pedestrians of the ambulance's presence. They also warn motorists approaching a stopped ambulance in a dangerous position on the road.

These warning lights commonly include flashing blue lights; strobes or LEDs fitted to the roof, front, sides and rear; and flashing headlights.

Blue flashing lights are only permitted to be used by services defined by the regulations that govern their use (the Road Vehicles Lighting Regulations 1989) – see Chapter 8 for more information on this.

In relation to the use of flashing headlights, many emergency vehicles have the facility to disable this type of warning from being activated at night when the vehicle headlights are switched on. This minimises the risk of dazzling other drivers.

Some Ambulance Trusts that serve the UK's airports may have airport beacons fitted to their emergency vehicles. These are yellow in colour and should only be used when the vehicle is deployed at the airport's 'airside'.

Audible warnings

Sirens

Most modern ambulances are fitted with electronic sirens that have the benefit of alerting people to the presence of an ambulance before they are able to see it. Sirens can usually produce a range of different noises that can be useful in different situations, for example:

- 'Wail' setting – characterised by a long up and down variation with an unbroken tone, the 'wail' setting can be used on a clear road approaching a junction.

- 'Yelp' setting – similar to the 'wail' setting but faster, the 'yelp' siren may be preferred in heavy slow traffic. It is less subject to sound deflection, which can cause confusion as to the direction of approach of the emergency vehicle.

- 'Dual-tone' sirens – these emit two different siren tones simultaneously, which can be beneficial when manoeuvring through heavy traffic or approaching junctions.

Ambulance Trusts may specifically train their drivers to use different siren tones in different situations, so refer to your local policy.

RDS systems

A recent development is the use of RDS (radio data system), the communication protocol that enables traffic broadcasts to be delivered to FM car radios within range.

Ambulances can be fitted with an FM transmitter set to RDS code 31, which enables them to interrupt the radio of all cars within range. Unlike traffic broadcasts, however, the user of the receiving radio is unable to opt out of the message (this feature is built into every RDS radio for broadcasts in case of a national emergency).

The use of short-range broadcast systems in emergency vehicles can be an effective means of alerting traffic to their proximity. The system is unlikely to replace sirens, however, as it is unable to alert those not using a compatible radio or other road users such as pedestrians.

Use of sirens when travelling in convoy

Where possible it is good practice to limit travelling in convoy while engaged under ERD. However, it is accepted within modern-day ambulance functions that this is not always possible, and sometimes unavoidable, especially at times of a serious or major incident or with the presence of rapid-response vehicles and specialist resilience vehicles such as the Hazardous Area Response Team (HART).

In this event, it is good practice to activate a different siren sound to the vehicle being followed and, in addition to this, the vehicles behind the lead vehicle need to be extra vigilant with regard to the unexpected behaviour of other traffic and the public, who may not be expecting more than one emergency vehicle.

Emergency warning equipment in practice

Drivers of emergency vehicles have a duty to warn other road users of their presence and intentions by exposing, to those who would benefit, any warning equipment (visual or audible) that is fitted to the vehicle. This should be balanced against the occasions when it offers more protection to deactivate audible warning equipment, for example when in standing traffic, to replace intimidation with invitation.

Blue flashing lights and sirens influence the behaviour of other road users; this is due to the presence of the emergency vehicle and the urgency of the journey being undertaken. They do not give any legal entitlement to claim unsafe precedence. You should also be aware at all times that if you have Emergency Warning Equipment fitted to a vehicle, the public have the right to receive the warning the equipment is designed to give.

The nature of loud sirens may be intimidating to others; they must be used intelligently in stationary traffic when there is a risk of threatening or forcing other vehicles to commit to a potentially dangerous manoeuvre that they may not have committed in the absence of the emergency vehicle. In this case, deactivation of the sirens must be considered.

In the event of a solo-response driver remaining with the patient en-route to the hospital (due to their advanced clinical skills, for example), one of the ambulance crew members may be asked to drive the solo-response vehicle (SRV) to the receiving hospital. When this situation arises, the SRV must not utilise Emergency Warning Equipment and must adhere to all road traffic regulations.

If you believe that the vehicle in front may not have heard the siren, changing the siren tone may gain their attention.

Knowledge recap questions

1. Describe an emergency vehicle's passive visual warnings.

2. Describe an emergency vehicle's active visual warnings.

3. Different siren tones can be beneficial in different situations. When might it be preferable to use a 'yelp' setting rather than a 'wail' setting?

4. Why is the RDS short-range broadcasting system unlikely to replace conventional sirens?

5. What is the best practice for the use of sirens should you find yourself travelling to an incident in convoy with other emergency response vehicles?

6. In what circumstances should the deactivation of sirens be considered and why?

8 Lighting Regulations

The Road Vehicles Lighting Regulations 1989 (and amendments made in 2005) set out all aspects of when and how motor vehicles should be lit on public roads. Drivers of emergency response vehicles must be aware of them, in particular the specific rules that apply to the use of emergency warning lights and their restrictions.

This chapter provides a summary of these regulations and their amendments, and links to the full legislation for further reading.

Learning outcomes

By the end of this chapter you should:

▲ Know the exceptional circumstances under which it is legal to have lights that are not in full working order.

▲ Know which vehicles may be fitted with a blue flashing light.

▲ Know when it is legally acceptable to use your blue flashing lights.

▲ Understand the amendments made to the Road Vehicles Lighting Regulations in 2005.

▲ Be able to access full versions of the Road Vehicles Lighting Regulations.

Road Vehicles Lighting Regulations 1989

The information provided in this chapter is a simplification of the Road Vehicles Lighting Regulations 1989 and the amendments made to them in 2005.

All lights must be clean and in full working order. The only exceptions to this are when:

- A light has stopped working on your current journey
- You have tried everything reasonable to fix it
- You are towing a trailer with working lights (so your vehicle's broken light cannot be seen).

In accordance with the Vehicles Lighting Regulations 1989, only emergency vehicles are permitted to have blue flashing lights or anything that resembles them, whether they are in working order or not. However, amendments to these regulations were made in 2005 (see below).

The only times that your blue flashing lights may be used are:

- When you are responding to an incident
- When you are at the scene of an incident
- To warn others of your approach or presence
- To let people know that there is a hazard on the road
- To facilitate the medical treatment of a patient with urgent need.

Changes made in 2005

In 2005 a number of changes were made to the lighting regulations. They can be summarised as follows:

1. Emergency vehicles are no longer defined as having to have a motor (for example, bicycles).

2. Anyone may use flashing lights on their bicycles (one to four flashes per second, with an equal amount of time on and off, in the usual colours).

3. Bicycles with lights attached to the wheels or in the pedals are now permitted.

4. HM Revenue & Customs may use blue flashing lights when investigating a serious crime.

5. Abnormal load escort vehicles are defined and permitted to use amber flashing lights when travelling at speeds above 25mph.

6. Authorised vehicle examiners may drive a vehicle on the road that does not have the correct lighting if it is going to, or returning from, a test, and they do not believe that the defects are dangerous.

Further reading

The full legislation on lighting is available on the legislation.gov.uk website, which is managed by The National Archives on behalf of the government. Drivers should remember that legislation is periodically updated and that it is their responsibility to keep up to date with any changes.

Links to the Road Vehicles Lighting Regulations are given below:

- Road Vehicles Lighting Regulations 1989:
  www.legislation.gov.uk/uksi/1989/1796/made

- Road Vehicles Lighting (Amendment) Regulations 2005:
  www. legislation.gov.uk/uksi/2005/2559/contents/made

- Road Vehicles Lighting (Amendment No. 2) Regulations 2005:
  www. legislation.gov.uk/uksi/2005/3169/contents/made

Knowledge recap questions

1. In which circumstances is it acceptable to have lights on a vehicle that are not in full working order?

2. Which vehicles may be fitted with blue flashing lights?

3. Name three situations in which the use of blue flashing lights is permitted.

9 Reversing and Manoeuvring

A significant percentage of collisions involving NHS Trust ambulance service vehicles occur while carrying out low-speed manoeuvres, especially those involving reversing. More collisions occur while reversing than in any other category.

Many, if not all, of these incidents could be avoided if basic standard procedures were diligently put into practice; often negligence has a major influence. This would significantly reduce repair costs and vehicle downtime, as well as promoting safety and reducing the risk of personal injury.

This chapter outlines the best practice procedures that should be employed when carrying out low-speed manoeuvres with an emphasis on the importance of teamwork.

Learning outcomes

By the end of this chapter you should:

▲ Know the rules and advice on reversing as specified in *The Highway Code*.

▲ Recognise the need for teamwork.

▲ Understand the driver's responsibilities when carrying out low-speed manoeuvres.

▲ Understand the attendant's or banksman's responsibilities when carrying out low-speed manoeuvres.

▲ Recognise and use the standard signals used to guide drivers when manoeuvring.

▲ Know not to solely rely on the use of proximity sensors and cameras when reversing.

Good theory and practice

The Highway Code sets out general rules and advice on reversing and manoeuvring for the benefit of all drivers. In addition, the following advice is given:

- Only turn the steering wheel while the vehicle is moving, thereby avoiding damage to the tyres, steering linkage and any power-assisted steering mechanisms.

- Utilise slow vehicle speed in conjunction with rapid hand movements on the steering wheel when manoeuvring in confined areas.

- Turn the steering wheel in the direction of the next vehicle movement just before ending the previous movement.

- Keep the vehicle moving slowly, controlling speed by engaging/disengaging the clutch or, in the case of automatic transmission, using the footbrake to control the speed.

- Carefully observe the front of the vehicle as it swings left or right while carrying out reversing turns.

- Consider using hazard warning lights to illuminate an area if reversing lights fail in conditions of reduced visibility.

- Avoid over-revving the engine, remembering that engine tickover may be sufficient on level ground.

The importance of teamwork

Very few, if any, reversing collisions occur when the correct standard procedure is followed, that is when an attendant or banksman is assisting the driver from the correct vantage point outside the vehicle. This vantage point should always be at the rear nearside (unless there are unusual circumstances that make this unsafe or impractical) as this is the point furthest away from the driver.

With the driver in the driving seat and the attendant at the rear nearside, responsibilities are shared as follows.

The driver is responsible for:

- Making sure that the attendant can be clearly seen in the nearside mirror before commencing the manoeuvre

- Controlling the speed of the vehicle

- Bringing the vehicle to an immediate halt if the attendant disappears from view

- Ensuring safety at the front and offside of the vehicle

- Ensuring any audible reverse warnings fitted are utilised.

The attendant is responsible for:

- Taking up a position at the rear nearside of the vehicle, in a position where they can be seen in the driver's nearside mirror

- Ensuring that their signals remain visible in the driver's nearside mirror by adjusting their position as the vehicle moves

- Ensuring safety at the rear and nearside of the vehicle, as well as roof clearance

- Ensuring that any audible reversing alarms fitted to the vehicle are active while the vehicle is in reverse.

> **REMEMBER!**
>
> It is vital that the attendant/banksman remains in the driver's view at all times. In the event of loss of view by the driver, the vehicle must be brought to an immediate standstill.

The driver and attendant should discuss and agree an appropriate plan before commencing the manoeuvre. It is important that standard, recognisable hand and arm signals are used (shown in Figure 9.1). These can be augmented by verbal signs – opening the nearside window will facilitate this.

If the major hazard is to the rear of the nearside, the driver should concentrate on following the attendant's signals, with occasional glances to the front of the vehicle and offside mirror to ensure safety. If the major

Reversing and Manoeuvring   **83**

hazard is to the front or offside, the driver should concentrate on these areas, with occasional glances in the nearside mirror to ensure safety.

The attendant must not stand in a position directly between a moving vehicle and a stationary object (such as a wall or another vehicle). Where it is impossible or impractical for the attendant to take up a position at the rear nearside, the best alternative should be adopted. Extra care should be taken in these circumstances.

Extra care should also be taken if an attendant is not on hand to assist. Consideration should be given to obtaining assistance if a suitable person is available. The driver has full responsibility for the safety of the manoeuvre in these circumstances.

The driver should consider winding down windows to enable verbal warnings to be heard.

A warning on using reverse sensors

Drivers should not rely entirely on the technology of audible reverse sensors or cameras (if fitted to their vehicle) as they can sometimes omit blind spots or certain parts of the vehicle. They should be considered as a reversing aid only!

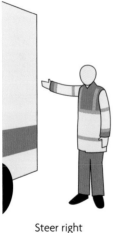

Steer right

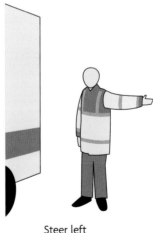

Steer left

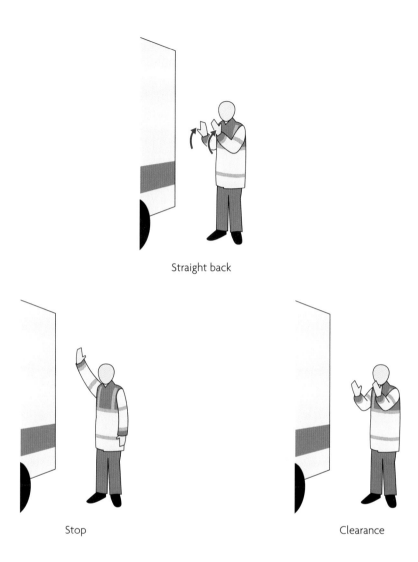

Straight back

Stop

Clearance

Figure 9.1   An attendant using arm and hand signals.

Knowledge recap questions

1. Why shouldn't the steering wheel be turned when the vehicle is stationary?

2. In what circumstances would it be appropriate to use hazard warning lights when carrying out low-speed manoeuvres?

3. What is the best position for an assisting attendant or banksman to stand in when a reversing manoeuvre is being carried out?

4. What action should be taken if an assisting attendant or banksman disappears from the driver's view while reversing?

5. What precautions should be taken when reversing if an attendant is not present or available?

6. Why should reverse sensors/cameras only be regarded as a reversing aid?

10 Attending Incidents

A consistent, uniform approach to attending incidents on motorways, dual carriageways and other roads by the emergency services is essential. This chapter outlines the best practice procedures described in *Practice Advice on the Policing of Roads*, a booklet produced by the National Policing Improvement Agency.

Topics covered include strategies to be used when approaching, parking at and leaving incidents on multi-lane carriageways and smaller roads, as well as specific procedures to be followed when you are the first emergency vehicle on scene, travelling in convoy or are accompanied by a police escort.

Dual carriageways may have many of the same characteristics of a motorway, such as hard shoulders, central reservations and speed limits. While their designations are different, the principles applied to motorways should equally be applied to dual carriageways.

Learning outcomes

By the end of this chapter you should:

▲ Understand the importance of personal protective equipment.

▲ Understand the importance of scene preservation at serious or fatal road traffic accidents.

▲ Know how to approach motorway or dual carriageway incidents when traffic is moving slowly or is stationary.

▲ Know the precautions that must be taken when driving on the hard shoulder.

By the end of this chapter you should:

▲ Know how to approach motorway or dual carriageway incidents when the carriageway is blocked or closed.

▲ Understand why travelling in convoy should be avoided and the precautions that must be taken when it is unavoidable.

▲ Know the safest position in which to park when attending incidents on the motorway or dual carriageway.

▲ Understand the importance of regular situation reports to ambulance control.

▲ Know the best practice procedures for leaving a scene.

▲ Know what to do if you come across an incident when driving a non-emergency vehicle for your Trust.

▲ Know the circumstances in which a police escort may be required and the procedure to follow.

Personal protective equipment

Personal protective equipment (PPE) – including a fastened high-visibility jacket and hard helmet – should be worn at every incident, no matter how minor it may seem. This is especially true when attending an incident on a motorway or dual carriageway. Serious head injuries can be and have been sustained by members of the emergency services who have been struck by objects thrown up by vehicles passing at high speeds.

Staff should decide whether any further protection is required when carrying out their risk assessment of the incident.

Scene preservation

It is important to remember that the scene of any serious or fatal road traffic accident is considered a crime scene by the police. Although it should not interfere with the care and treatment of patients, which is paramount, you should be mindful when on scene to minimise the unnecessary disturbance of potential evidence.

Motorways and multi-lane carriageways

Approach

The high volume of vehicles on motorways and dual carriageways and the speeds at which they travel present ambulance staff with unique problems. Minor incidents can rapidly expand to involve a large number of vehicles, while any incident may lead to a large build-up of traffic, causing difficulties for approaching emergency response vehicles.

Different methods of approaching incidents on multi-lane carriageways have been devised depending on the traffic conditions.

Flowing traffic

Ambulances should approach using the main carriageway whenever possible, usually in lanes two or three (see Figure 10.1). This allows other road users to react in a normal manner, moving left when seeing an approaching ambulance or hearing sirens. Do not use lane one – this could cause drivers to move onto the hard shoulder where other vehicles may have stopped.

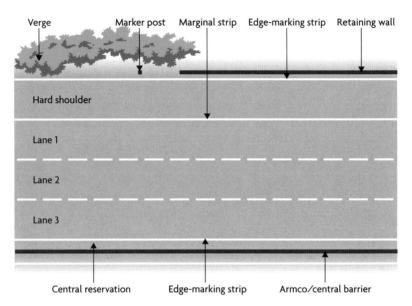

Figure 10.1 Layout of a motorway.

Completely blocked: slow-moving or stationary traffic

If the road is completely blocked by slow-moving or stationary traffic, you will need to approach using the hard shoulder. Depending on the conditions of the traffic on the main carriageway, different strategies should be employed:

- **Traffic on the main carriageway is moving slowly:** approach on the hard shoulder with only visual warning equipment activated (blue lights and flashing headlights). Do not use sirens. The use of sirens has been known to cause drivers to pull onto the hard shoulder, into the path of emergency response vehicles. You can use your normal road horn to indicate your presence if required.

- **Traffic on the main carriageway is stationary:** approach on the hard shoulder with all Emergency Warning Equipment activated – blue flashing lights and sirens. However, you must be aware of the danger of members of the public being on the hard shoulder – people sometimes get out of their vehicles to see what's going on or to stretch their legs if they have been in stationary traffic for some time.

Extreme caution is required when driving on the hard shoulder. The surface may have loose grit, oil and other objects present on it that would not normally be found on the main carriageway. Vehicles may be parked on the hard shoulder and, if broken down, may not have lights at night. People walking to or from emergency telephones may also pose a hazard. Your speed must be chosen with due regard for the circumstances.

Blockage or closure

The police may direct drivers to turn around and drive back to the previous exit if an incident has led to the complete blockage or closure of the motorway. You will be notified by the police at the junction where vehicles are being directed off the road if this is taking place. The normal rules of the road apply in these circumstances:

- Drive in lane one, on the left; do not use the hard shoulder
- Use visual warning equipment (blue lights and flashing headlights)
- Keep your speed down.

Any traffic that has been turned around by the police will be kept to their left, in single file and at a slow speed.

The police may also direct you to approach or leave an incident in the wrong direction if the carriageway is blocked or closed. In these circumstances the same procedure applies:

- Drive on the left
- Use visual warning equipment (blue lights and flashing headlights)
- Keep your speed down
- Be aware that other emergency response vehicles may be travelling towards you on the same carriageway.

Follow the instructions of police officers at all times. Highways Agency support staff may also be required to direct traffic control (see Appendix 3).

Travelling in convoy

Emergency response vehicles travelling under emergency conditions (with visual and audible warnings activated) should try to avoid travelling in convoy. Other road users may be unable to clearly identify the number of vehicles approaching and may not expect more than one emergency vehicle.

If the situation requires a number of vehicles to travel to the same incident, however, consideration should be given to an appropriate distance being maintained between vehicles and to the choice of siren used (see Chapter 7).

Parking

Crews must perform a risk assessment when arriving on scene, taking the directions of other staff or agencies already present into account to ensure their own safety.

Parking at a scene already protected by the police or other agency

Ambulances should park at the front of the incident within the coned-off area (see Figure 10.2) if the scene is already protected by the police or another agency, such as the fire and rescue service or Highways Agency.

Blue lights and flashing headlights should be turned off when parked within the safe area – doing so significantly reduces the risks arising from 'rubbernecking' motorists. Police vehicles, which should be parked at the rear of the scene, will provide rear-facing blue and red lights.

> ### REMEMBER!
> If you are the first emergency vehicle to arrive at a scene, remember that your own safety is paramount. A full risk assessment must be undertaken.

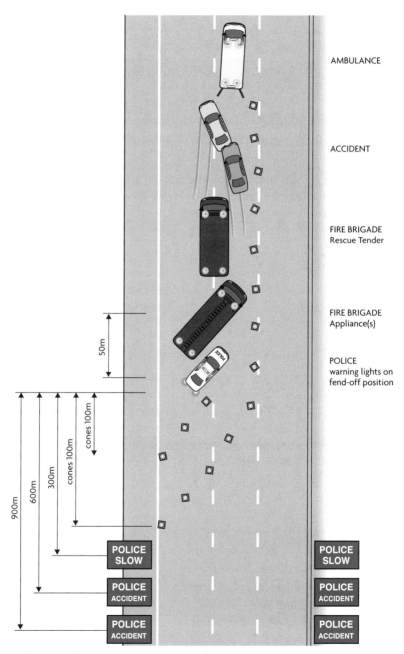

AMBULANCE

ACCIDENT

FIRE BRIGADE
Rescue Tender

FIRE BRIGADE
Appliance(s)

POLICE
warning lights on
fend-off position

50m

cones 100m

cones 100m

cones 100m

300m

600m

900m

POLICE
SLOW

POLICE
ACCIDENT

POLICE
ACCIDENT

POLICE
SLOW

POLICE
ACCIDENT

POLICE
ACCIDENT

Figure 10.2   Parking in a coned-off area.

First emergency vehicle on scene – incidents confined to the hard shoulder

The following parking procedure should be followed when you are the first emergency vehicle arriving at an unprotected scene on the hard shoulder:

- Stop 50m before the incident in a straight line with the carriageway.

- If there is no physical barrier or other obstruction (such as a bridge support) turn the front wheels towards the nearside; if there is a barrier turn the front wheels outwards towards the carriageway. If the vehicle is subsequently struck from behind, it will then be steered away from you rather than pushed straight towards the incident you are attending.

- Switch off forward-facing blue lights and flashing headlights, but keep on your rear-facing blue and/or red lights (if fitted), sidelights and hazard lights. Keeping the rear doors closed when not required to be open will ensure that their reflective, high-visibility markings can be seen.

If possible, stay behind the barrier when walking towards the incident. If this is not possible, stay as far away from the live carriageway as you can. Keep your eye on approaching traffic.

Local procedures

Some local police authorities advocate that emergency vehicles attending motorway or dual carriageway incidents leave all their visual warnings activated. Drivers should be guided by their local Trust's policy.

First emergency vehicle on scene – incidents in lanes one, two or three, or a combination

If you are first on scene at an incident on the main carriageways, you may need to place your vehicle in a **fend-off** position – refer to your local Trust's procedures. This extremely hazardous position involves using the vehicle to block one or more lanes, and should be performed with the utmost caution.

Stop 50m back from the incident, turning the front wheels in a safe direction to reduce the risk of the vehicle being pushed into the incident if it is struck. You should also stop in a position that affords maximum visibility of rear visual devices and reflective/high-visibility markings; all rear-facing visual warnings – blue lights, rear-flashing red lights, sidelights, fog lights and hazard lights – should be activated.

- Fending off lane one – park at a slight angle but do not intrude into lane two.

- Fending off lane two – park at an angle to obstruct lanes one and two but do not intrude into lane three.

- Fending off lane three – park at a slight angle but do not intrude into lane two.

- Fending off lanes two and three – park at an angle to obstruct lanes two and three but do not intrude into lane one.

The police will permit you to block as many lanes as required to ensure your own safety and that of your patients.

No one should return to the ambulance once it is parked in a fend-off position unless absolutely necessary.

Keep your eye on passing traffic; you must never assume it is safe. Research has shown that a significant proportion of drivers are unable to distinguish a stationary vehicle on a motorway or dual carriageway from one that is moving.

See Appendix 1 for details on parking high-dependency service (HDS) and patient transport service (PTS) vehicles, and cars for service officers and BASICS doctors at incidents on motorways and dual carriageways.

Key term

Fend-off position – using your vehicle to block one or more lanes when attending an incident on the main carriageway of a motorway or multi-lane road.

Situation reports

If you are the first emergency vehicle on scene you should provide control with a situation report (SITREP) as soon as possible. It should contain the following information:

- Your location – the nearest marker post will confirm your location to within one-tenth of a kilometre (see Figure 10.3)

- Your direction of travel, for example northbound/southbound

- The number and types of vehicles involved in the incident

- Which lanes of the carriageway are involved

- Whether any hazardous loads are involved.

This information will be passed on to the police or Highways Agency control – they will activate the matrix signs, if available, to warn approaching motorists.

Key term

SITREP – situation report provided to control detailing your exact location, direction of travel, number and type of vehicles involved in the incident, number of casualties and whether further assistance is required.

Figure 10.3 Example of a marker post. The figures are a distance in kilometres from a defined point and will give your location within 100m. This post is 25.3km from the defined point.

You must keep control regularly informed. Subsequent SITREPs should include:

- The number of casualties

- The types of injuries sustained

- Requests for further vehicles if required

- Requests for air ambulance if required (see Appendix 2)

- Whether assistance is required from other agencies, for example the fire and rescue service

- Notifying hospitals.

Leaving the scene

Rejoining moving traffic when leaving the incident scene is also extremely hazardous – other road users may be too busy 'rubbernecking' to notice that you are moving.

If there is a clear path in front of you, you should proceed in a straight line in that lane or on the hard shoulder. You can change lanes when you have built up enough speed to match the traffic conditions around you. Your rear blue lights should remain activated until you have rejoined the normal traffic flow; you can then turn them off if not conveying patients to hospital as an emergency.

You will require the assistance of a police officer or Highways Agency traffic officer if your path is obstructed. Build up speed quickly to match the traffic around you; you can then turn off your blue lights unless they are required for your journey.

Other urban and rural roads

Attending the scene of an incident on any road, including those in residential areas, presents a degree of risk. Emergency response crews should not become complacent and should be especially aware of the risks associated with 'red mist' – paying too much attention to what *may* be presented at the scene before arriving at it can allow intrusive thoughts to influence your decision-making process. Regardless of the medical competencies or skills the clinician may have, these hold no value until such time as safe arrival on scene has taken place.

As with motorways and dual carriageways, stopping on any high-speed road – or indeed anywhere where other vehicular activity is present – is potentially high risk, especially for covert vehicles that may be attending these incidents.

Non-emergency vehicles at scenes

Other vehicles that operate within the Trust, for example PTS vehicles, may periodically come across incidents on highways and may not be fitted with the appropriate Emergency Warning Equipment. In these instances, the driver should perform a dynamic risk assessment and consider whether it may be safer to park away from the incident and provide control with a SITREP rather than to stop at the scene.

This can be very difficult, but you must not be tempted to put yourself in danger except in case of the immediate preservation of life. See Appendix 1 for further information on non-emergency vehicles attending motorway or dual carriageway incidents.

Stopping and parking at the scene

When parking at the scene of any emergency, crew and vehicle safety must be paramount. Parking should, where possible, take place in an area that facilitates safe egress for staff, minimising the danger caused by passing vehicles.

Consideration should be given to the likelihood of patient loading, such as the clearance required for ramps and tail lifts. If the vehicle is parked partly on the pavement, this may mean that the ramp or tail lift may not deploy correctly due to the kerb impeding its operation.

The use of warning lights should be appropriate for the density of hazards present or potentially present. In residential areas the use of hazard warning lights alone may be sufficient, whereas other rural or urban roads may require the full use of emergency warning lighting.

When parking at night ensure that, as a minimum, the vehicle sidelights are illuminated, particularly if you have to park facing oncoming traffic.

Solo responders need to consider the most appropriate parking positions carefully, particularly in residential areas. Parking directly outside a private dwelling to attend to a patient may inconvenience any following back-up vehicle when they need to park and load a patient.

Consider:

- Initial mobile reconnaissance or dynamic risk assessment. Which parking option offers the maximum protection? Is there a safer alternative? Review regularly.

- PPE must always be put on prior to leaving the vehicle.

- Consider unseen or unheard vehicle activity that may be hidden in the blind spot of the vehicle on the side from which you are exiting.

- What warning equipment is fitted to your vehicle that could provide greater protection?

- The activation of rear red flashing lights is very effective due to their primary colour attraction; however, in the presence of mist or fog this can be distracting for other vehicles, which may not see you initially. Look, listen and be extremely vigilant about the potential of developing hazards as yet unseen.

Police escorts

Occasionally circumstances may dictate that an ambulance requires a police escort on its journey, for example if it is vital that the journey to hospital is a slow, uninterrupted and smooth one, or that the journey time is reduced. This request must usually be approved by ambulance control (refer to your local Trust's procedures). The police will provide an escort if they are in agreement that one will indeed cut the journey time or make it slower and safer, and if police resources are available.

The following procedure for escorts given by police motorcycles or other police vehicles has been offered by members of the Police Driver Standards Group:

- One is positioned at the front of the ambulance, and it is their role to maintain a safe and constant speed.

- Another is positioned on the offside of the ambulance, visible in the ambulance's offside wing mirror.

- The final motorcycle is positioned to block off traffic at the next major hazard, such as a junction or a roundabout.

- As the ambulance goes through the hazard, the bike controlling the hazard takes up a position on the offside of the ambulance. The bike that was previously in this position moves up to control the next hazard.

Alternative procedures are in operation around the country, and it is in the interests of all services to work across boundaries and within written local policies and procedures.

There is no exemption or entitlement for an ambulance solo responder to provide an escort for another emergency ambulance vehicle with emergency warning equipment activated under any circumstances. This is a specialised function and must not be undertaken by persons untrained or unauthorised.

Knowledge recap questions

1. Explain why personal protective equipment is essential when attending incidents on a multi-lane carriageway.

2. What is 'scene preservation' and why is it important?

3. Which lanes should be used when approaching an incident on a motorway or dual carriageway in flowing traffic?

4. What precautions should be taken when approaching an incident on a motorway or dual carriageway by driving on the hard shoulder?

5. Explain why sirens should not be used when approaching an incident on a motorway by driving on the hard shoulder if the traffic on the main carriageway is moving slowly.

6. Why should a number of emergency vehicles responding to a single incident avoid travelling in a convoy?

7. Where is the correct place to park at an incident on a motorway or dual carriageway that is already being attended by another emergency service?

8. What is a 'fend-off' parking position and when would you use it?

9. What information should be relayed to control in an initial situation report (SITREP)?

10. What information should be relayed to control in subsequent SITREPs?

11. Describe the procedure for leaving the scene of an incident on the motorway or dual carriageway if the path ahead of you is clear.

12. What procedure should you follow if you come across an incident while driving a vehicle that is not fitted with emergency warning equipment?

13. In what circumstances might you request a police escort?

14. Can an ambulance solo responder provide an escort for another emergency ambulance vehicle in some circumstances?

11 Eco-Driving

Eco-driving is a term used to describe smarter and more fuel-efficient driving. While it is accepted that the nature of ERD is not always conducive to eco-driving due to the driving principles and systems engaged, there are arguably many occasions when ambulance service vehicles drive under normal conditions and, therefore, every effort should be made to help to reduce the carbon footprint of the service.

This chapter outlines the ways in which emergency response drivers can reduce their fuel consumption by driving in the most energy-efficient way when not driving under emergency response conditions.

Learning outcomes

By the end of this chapter you should:

▲ Understand what eco-driving means.

▲ Know the techniques that can be used to drive in a more environmentally (and economically) friendly way when not employing ERD procedures.

Economical driving

Driving in a way that gets the most out of the fuel in your vehicle not only cuts down on greenhouse gas emissions and other pollutants, it also reduces costs. When not driving under emergency response conditions, drivers of NHS Trust vehicles have a responsibility to contribute positively to this.

The AA offers the following advice on fuel and the environment:

- Accelerate gently and smoothly – this can be aided by the accurate use of driving plans and good acceleration sense.

- Decelerate smoothly and early for hazards or in preparation to stop.

- Keep the vehicle rolling wherever possible – moving off from being stationary uses more fuel.

- Change gear early so as not to labour the engine. An rpm of 2000 in a diesel vehicle is often a good engine speed to indicate a gear change; alternatively, respond to the gear shift indicator light if fitted.

- Try to reduce the use of the air conditioning system at low speeds; this tends to use more fuel (less noticeable at higher speeds). On a warm day open windows to create air flow.

- Electrical load increases fuel consumption. Turn off demister blowers and lights when not required.

- Comply with posted speed limits. The faster the speed, the greater the fuel consumption and, therefore, pollution. Travelling at 80mph can use up to 25% more fuel than travelling at 70mph.

- While stationary in a queue of traffic, consider switching the engine off for delays of more than three minutes.

Knowledge recap questions

1. What does 'eco-driving' mean?

2. What are the benefits of driving in a more fuel-efficient way?

3. Describe three techniques that can be used to drive in a more environmentally friendly way.

Appendices

Appendix 1: HDS, PTS, officers' cars and BASICS doctors attending incidents on motorways and dual carriageways

HDS and PTS staff must not attend incidents on motorways or dual carriageways without the correct PPE.

High Dependency Service (HDS) vehicles

HDS vehicles must only be sent to an incident on a motorway or multi-lane carriageway if the presence of a safe coned-off area has been confirmed; they should park within this coned area following the same arrangements as other emergency vehicles.

HDS vehicles must not be used in fend-off positions if they have inadequate emergency warning lights or markings (refer to your local Trust's policy).

Patient Transport Service (PTS) vehicles

PTS vehicles should only attend incidents if the motorway has been closed or a safe coned-off area has been confirmed. They should then follow the same parking arrangements as other emergency and utility vehicles.

Like HDS vehicles, PTS vehicles must not be used in fend-off positions if they do not have emergency lights or suitable markings.

Officers' and BASICS doctors' cars

Officers' cars and BASICS doctors' cars should park in the coned-off area, towards the front, making sure that they do not block the exit of other emergency vehicles.

They must not be used in fend-off positions.

HDS, PTS, officers' cars and BASICS doctors arriving first on scene

If these vehicles arrive first at the scene of an incident or come across one, they should:

- Switch on any visual warnings available

- Park in front of the incident

- Contact control with an initial SITREP

- Perform a dynamic risk assessment – if the situation is unsafe they should remain in their vehicle.

Do not approach an incident until a safe coned-off area has been established. This can be very difficult, but you must not be tempted to put yourself in danger, except in case of the immediate preservation of life.

Appendix 2: Air ambulance

You must inform the police officers on scene at the earliest opportunity if you need to request the attendance of an air ambulance. Ambulance control will contact police or Highways Agency control centres to confirm that the air ambulance will be attending.

Additional police officers may be required as the motorway or dual carriageway will have to be closed in both directions if the air ambulance intends to land on the road. For the same reasons, let police officers at the scene know as soon as possible if control informs you that they have mobilised the air ambulance.

Appendix 3: Highways Agency Traffic Officers

Highways Agency Traffic Officers (HATOs) will lead in the management of incidents in which there is no injury or alleged offence to:

- Deal with congestion

- Ensure the safe and speedy removal of obstructions
- Assist vulnerable road users.

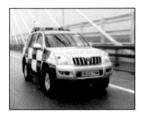

Figure A3.1   HATO vehicle.

The police will maintain scene control for any incidents that involve:

- Death
- Injury
- Criminality
- Threats to public order and safety
- Major coordination of emergency responders.

Powers granted to HATOs

HATOs' powers are detailed in the Traffic Management Act 2004. Section 4 sets out the legal relationship between HATOs and the police, and states that:

1. When carrying out their duties a HATO shall comply with any direction of a police officer.

2. Subject to that, when carrying out their duties a HATO, when designated by an authorised person, shall comply with any direction of the appropriate national authority.

Ambulance staff should note that HATOs have restricted powers. They are only trained to deal with the following situations on the road network:

- Maintaining or improving the flow of traffic
- Preventing or reducing congestion

- Avoiding danger to persons or traffic, or the risk of such danger occurring
- Preventing damage to anything on or near the road.

The main powers granted to HATOs are the authority to:
- Stop or direct traffic, including cyclists and rolling road blocks
- Direct vehicles for traffic surveys
- Direct persons on foot
- Place temporary traffic signs.

On the arrival of ambulance staff, HATOs will look to give an update on the number, age, gender and injuries of the casualties. They will also ask if any further safety measures are required, such as additional lane closures.

HATOs have a responsibility to the regional control centres for strategic roads and will need to know the number of casualties requiring treatment and what hospital they will be taken to. A basic state of injury will also be required.

Appendix 4: Driving commentary

Emergency response drivers are trained in the technique of driving commentary – giving a running verbal commentary on what they can see, what they predict might happen and what action they intend to do take.

The reasons for giving a commentary while driving are:
1. To help drivers cultivate distant and/or detailed observations
2. To develop logical reasoning and planning
3. To assist driving instructors to assess students' powers of observation and lines of reasoning along with hazard prioritisation.

Introduction
1. Type of area
2. Speed limit
3. Weather conditions
4. Traffic volume.

Examples

I'm driving on a single carriageway road with one lane in each direction. The road is divided by central lane markings, the surface is dry and is conducive to firm braking. It's a residential area with a speed limit of 30mph...

The object is to form a 'word picture' of the changing scene around the vehicle. The description should include:

1. Identification of any hazards

2. Action to be taken

3. Reasons for that action.

Points regarding system application should be included where appropriate and when convenient. It is most important that all comments in relation to identifying hazards and the action contemplated are concluded (see Table A4.1).

Table A4.1 Commentary examples for specific hazards.

Feature	Reasoning and driving actions
Garage forecourt on nearside	Clear, no danger or vehicles present. I am slowing down and/or moving out, increasing the margin of safety.
Ice cream van parked on offside	Unattended, no danger or children present, reducing speed, taking a lower gear.
Crossroads ahead, I have priority	Open or blind. I will take centre-line position to minimise danger from the nearside.
Warning sign ahead	Bend to the offside. Check mirrors, adjust my vehicle position and approach speed to negotiate the bend, watching the limit point.

Table A4.1 Commentary examples for specific hazards. *continued*

Feature	Reasoning and driving actions
School sign	Bearing in mind the time of day, day of week, month of year, are there children about?
Cattle sign	I will keep a sharp lookout because animals tend to wander out in front of traffic.
Light is poor	I will use dipped headlamps to see and be seen. I will show extreme caution. Bad light affects vision, including pedestrians.

Try to imagine that the person for whom you are commentating cannot see and has no idea where you are, what you are doing and why you are doing it. It is your task to outline events as they occur as fully as your speed and commitments allow, satisfying all safety aspects.

A commentary that cannot be heard is a wasted effort. Speak up, particularly when travelling at high speed, when the combined noises of wind, tyre suction, engine and transmission make it difficult for you to be heard.

Commentary on the system

It is important that you learn the five phases of the system of car control and put them into operation. Try doing this for hazards such as traffic lights, major junctions, obstructions and where you intend to turn. Now you have to fill in the spaces between the systems, and for this you need a good knowledge of *The Highway Code*.

Five-phases system of car control

Roadcraft outlines a five-phase system of vehicle control: 'a way of approaching and negotiating hazards that is methodical, safe and leaves nothing to chance'. A hazard is defined as any potentially dangerous situation encountered.

The five phases are:

- **Information** – the driver's observations on what is going on around them, the actions they plan to make and the information they provide to other road users
- **Position** – confirming that the safest position on the road is being used for the circumstances
- **Speed** – braking or accelerating smoothly to an appropriate speed for the hazard being approached
- **Gear** – selecting the appropriate gear for optimum vehicle control
- **Acceleration** – smooth acceleration, clearing the hazard safely.

Spot commentaries can be particularly useful to help develop your prioritisation skills or to help improve observation links that may be deficient. These types of commentaries, as the name suggests, focus on particular areas of driving, which may include:

- Information signs
- Road markings
- Limit points
- New view information
- Junction activity.

Some examples of this follow below.

System of car control

I am driving the vehicle to the system of car control. This way of approaching and negotiating hazards is safe, methodical and leaves nothing to chance. It is a systematic way of dealing with an unpredictable and potentially dangerous environment.

System commentary for a hazard

Ahead now I see a direction sign indicating a crossroads. I intend to turn left and travel towards Cardiff. Before each phase of the system I shall take, use and give information. Mirror, I am already in position. Mirror, I am signalling to the vehicle behind and I am adjusting my speed. Having got the correct speed I am selecting a suitable gear. I am checking my mirror again and accelerating away from the hazard.

Hazards

A hazard is anything that is an actual or potential danger. On the road I could meet physical hazards, such as junctions and variations in road surfaces, or those caused by weather conditions, for example icy roads or poor visibility.

Reduction in speed limit

Ahead now I see speed restriction signs for 30mph. I check the mirror and the speedometer and reduce the speed by acceleration sense to the maximum permitted speed as I pass the signs.

Acceleration sense

I am reducing speed by acceleration sense. This is the ability to use the accelerator accurately to vary the vehicle's speed in response to changing road and traffic conditions.

Principles of cornering

As I negotiate the bend or corner, you will see that my vehicle is in the correct position. I am travelling at an appropriate speed; I am in the right gear; I am able to stop safely within the distance that I can see to be clear.

Double white lines

This section of the road is controlled by a system of double white lines with a continuous line on my side of the road. I must not straddle or cross it unless I need to pass something stationary in the road, to turn right in or out of premises or a junction, on the direction of a traffic warden or police officer owing to circumstances beyond my control, to avoid an accident or to pass another road user who is travelling at less than 10mph.

Zones

Ahead now the road disappears into a zone of invisibility. I divide the road into zones – zones of visibility, zones of invisibility, zones of safety and zones of danger – remembering that a zone of invisibility is a potential zone of danger and that I must not accelerate into these zones.

Advantages of correct steering technique

You will notice that adopting the correct steering technique provides safe and efficient steering in a wide range of circumstances; it enables me to turn the wheel immediately in either direction.

The 'lurker'

There is a large vehicle approaching; I am looking for the 'lurker' – the fast car or motorcycle that closes up behind such vehicles and then swoops out into view.

Following position

I am moving up into a following position. By keeping at the proper distance from the vehicle in front, I will gain the following advantages:

- *I will be able to maintain a good view, which can be increased along the nearside or offside by a very slight deviation, so that I can always be aware of what is happening in the immediate vicinity.*

- *I can stop the vehicle safely in the event of the driver in front braking firmly without warning.*

- *I can extend my braking distance so that a following driver is given more time in which to react.*

- *I can move up into an overtaking position when it is safe to do so and I will suffer less from the effects of spray from the vehicle in front.*

Appendix 5: Speed and safety

The following is a talk by Mr Justice Blair reported in the *Journal of Criminal Law* in 1988:

The basic cause of road accidents is widespread ignorance of ground speed, not only on the part of pedestrians but also on the part of virtually every driver of a motor car, and I add that if this widespread ignorance on the part of the road users be cured, and it is curable, then there will follow a great reduction in the toll of road accidents.

A speedometer does not tell anyone his ground speed. It does nothing of the kind, and it is because every motorist deludes himself into believing that a speedometer tells him how fast he is covering the ground that the danger of road accidents is increased. A speedometer gives you your speed in miles per hour. Have you any mental picture of the length of any hour or the length of a mile? No one has. How then can anyone possibly get a mental picture of his ground speed when he is asked to put two unreliable factors together and obtain a result?

I have tried very many running down cases. Judges are conscientious when trying cases and I always felt that in order to understand any motor case it was necessary that I work out a respective speed of each vehicle in a measure that would tell me their respective ground speeds. The only measure that would give me any mental picture of the speed at which a vehicle covered the ground was the measure of feet per second. That involved me in a lot of arithmetic. Sixty miles per hour works out at 87.9 recurring feet per second, and every time I converted miles per hour into feet per second I got a result in recurring decimals. So then I had to look for a simple formula, and this is how I got it.

Instead of calling 60mph, 87 odd feet per second, I called it 90 feet per second, and that gave me the simple formula of adding half to my miles per hour to obtain speed in feet per second correct within 2%. Ever since then, I have driven cars and tried running down cases in feet per second. Now what I say to all motorists is that they try doing what I do; that is, always to drive and think of speed in feet per second instead of in miles per hour, and you will at once become a 100% better and safer driver. All you have to do is to add one half to the figure of your speed in mph and you will get your speed in feet per second.

Any child can do that. The other aspect of road safety touches what is called kinetic energy, which means the moving force possessed by a vehicle in motion. I can't give you a more detailed explanation but another way to put it is to refer to kinetic energy as the kick possessed by a moving vehicle. A small motor car weighing about a ton and moving at a speed of 40mph strikes the same blow as 18 ten-ton steam rollers travelling at their highest speed, which is 3mph. That is the force you are handling when you speed a light car up to 40mph, 60 feet per second. If you are driving a big seven-seater, two-ton car at 60mph (90 feet per second) its kinetic energy is more than that of 100 ten-ton steam rollers moving at 3mph.

Unhappily, human nature is such that, when travelling from one place to another, drivers are all inspired with the same desire: to get to a destination as soon as possible, travelling as fast as possible, the controls comprised by the word 'possible' being (1) regard for your safety, (2) road sense, (3) consideration for others and (4) the law.

Consideration of 'feet per second' and 'kinetic energy' (see Table A5.1) do not occur to most of us until after an accident.

Table A5.1   Justice Blair's theory.

Feet per sec	Metres per sec	Miles per hour	Multiplier	Braking distance		Thinking distance		Overall stopping	
				Feet	Metres	Feet	Metres	Feet	Metres
45	13.73	30	1.5	45	13.73	30	9.15	75	22.88
60	18.30	40	2	80	24.40	40	12.20	120	36.60
75	22.88	50	2.5	125	38.13	50	15.25	175	53.38
90	27.45	60	3	180	54.90	60	18.30	240	73.20
105	32.03	70	3.5	245	74.73	70	21.35	315	96.08
120	36.60	80	4	320	97.60	80	24.40	400	122.00
135	41.18	90	4.5	405	123.53	90	27.45	495	150.98
150	45.75	100	5	500	152.50	100	30.50	600	183.00
165	50.33	110	5.5	605	184.53	110	33.55	715	218.08
180	54.90	120	6	720	219.60	120	36.60	840	256.20
195	59.48	130	6.5	845	257.73	130	39.65	975	297.38
210	64.05	140	7	980	298.90	140	42.70	1120	341.60
225	68.63	150	7.5	1125	343.13	150	45.75	1275	388.88
240	73.20	160	8	1280	390.40	160	48.80	1440	439.20
255	77.78	170	8.5	1445	440.73	170	51.85	1615	492.58
270	82.35	180	9	1620	494.10	180	54.90	1800	549.00
285	86.93	190	9.5	1805	550.53	190	57.95	1995	608.48
300	91.50	200	10	2000	610.00	200	61.00	2200	671.00

Knowledge recap questions

1. Is it possible to use high-dependency service and patient transport service vehicles in a fend-off position when attending incidents on a multi-lane carriageway?

2. What procedure should high-dependency service and patient transport service vehicles follow if they are first to arrive at the scene of an incident?

3. What procedure should you follow if you need to request the attendance of an air ambulance?

4. Why are emergency response drivers trained in the technique of driving commentary?

5. Describe the five phases of the system of car control.

Glossary

AACE	Association of Ambulance Chief Executives
ABS	Antilock Brake System
ASR	Acceleration Skid Control
BAS	Brake Assist System
BASICS	British Association for Immediate Care Schemes
COP	Codes of Practice
DTAG	Driver Training Advisory Group
DVLA	Driver and Vehicle Licensing Agency
EBD	Electronic Brakeforce Distribution
ERD	Emergency Response Driving
ESP	Electronic Stability Programme
EWE	Emergency Warning Equipment
HART	Hazardous Area Response Team
HATO	Highways Agency Traffic Officer
HDS	High-Dependency Service
HSDT	High Speed Driving Training
LGV	Large Goods Vehicle
PCV	Passenger Carrying Vehicle
PDC	Pre-Driving Check
PPE	Personal Protective Equipment
PTS	Patient Transport Service
RDS	Radio Data System
SITREP	Situation Report
SRD	Solo-Response Driver
SRV	Solo-Response Vehicle
VDI	Vehicle Daily Inspection

References

Ambulance Today, available at: www.ambulancetoday.co.uk/downloads/fleet_examples.pdf

Association of Chief Police Officers of England, Wales and Northern Ireland (2007) *Guidance regarding the legal obligations placed on forces as body corporate when dealing with speeding and red light offences by emergency service vehicles.* London: ACPO.

Blair, Mr Justice (1988) Speech reproduced in *Journal of Criminal Law*, 5 (January).

British Standards Institution (2010) *Medical vehicles and their equipment. Road ambulances.* BS EN 1789:2007+A1:2010. London: BSi.

Cook, S., Quigley, C. and Clift, L. (2000) *Motor vehicle and pedal cycle conspicuity – Part 1: Vehicle mounted warning beacons.* London: Department for Transport.

De Lorenzo, R.A. and Eilers, M.A. (1991) 'Lights and siren: a review of emergency vehicle warning systems', *Annals of Emergency Medicine*, 20(12), pp. 1331–5.

Dorn, L. (2013) *A behavioural analysis of fleet driver safety*, Driver Metrics blog post, 28 May 2013. Available at: www.drivermetrics.com/2013/05/behavioural-analysis-fleet-driver-safety

Heyward, B., Stanley, L. and Ward, N.J. (2009) *Risk-Seeking Behaviors and Emergency Medical Service Crash Risk in Rural Ambulance Drivers.* University Transportation Centers Program.

HMSO (2007) *The Highway Code.* Available at: www.gov.uk/browse/driving/highway-code

Ho, J. and Casey, B. (1998) 'Time saved with use of emergency warning lights and sirens during response to requests for emergency medical aid in an urban environment', *Annals of Emergency Medicine*, 32(5), pp. 585–8.

Ho, J. and Lindquist, M. (2001) 'Time saved with the use of emergency warning lights and siren while responding to requests for emergency medical aid in a rural environment', *Prehospital Emergency Care*, 5(2), pp. 159–62.

Howard, C.Q., Maddern, A.J. and Privopoulos, E.P. (2011) 'Acoustic characteristics for effective ambulance sirens', *Acoustics Australia*, 39(2), pp. 43–53.

Institute of Advanced Motorists (2011) *Licensed to Skill: Contributory Factors in Accidents*. London: Institute of Advanced Motorists.

Joint Emergency Service High Speed Driver Training Advisory Group (2008) *Provision of High Speed Driver Training Code of Practice*. Available at: www.gov.uk/government/uploads/system/uploads/attachment_data/file/162 65/high-speed-driver-training-2008.pdf

Lacher, M.E. and Bausher, J.C. (1997) 'Lights and siren in pediatric 911 ambulance transports: are they being misused?', *Annals of Emergency Medicine*, 29(2), pp. 223–7.

Mares, P., Coyne, P. and MacDonald, B. (2013) Roadcraft: *The Police Driver's Handbook*. Norwich: The Stationery Office.

Mercedes Benz (2014) *Sprinter operator manual edition MY*, pp. 32, 56, 57, 59, 60, 138–47, 151, 152, 156, 160, 172, 206–8, 221.

National Policing Improvement Agency (2007) *Practice Advice on the Policing of Roads*. National Policing Improvement Agency and the Association of Chief Police Officers.

Priestman, R. (2005) *Driver behaviour within the ambulance service: an exploratory study on driver behaviour, collision attribution and driving-related stressors*. Cranfield: Cranfield University School of Engineering.

Sharp, G., Seagar, H. and George, C. (1997) *Human Aspects of Police Driving*. Road Safety Scotland.

Withington, D. (2000) 'The use of directional sound to improve the safety of auditory warnings', *Proceedings of the Human Factors and Ergonomics Society Annual Meeting July 2000*, 44(22), pp. 726–9.

www.rospa.com/roadsafety/adviceandinformation/driving/automatic-gearboxes.aspx

Zachariah, B.S., Pepe, P.E., Persse, D.E. and Curka, P.A. (1994) 'The effect of warning lights and sirens on EMS response intervals', *Annals of Emergency Medicine*, 23(3), p. 637.

http://www.iam.org.uk/images/stories/policy-research/licensetoskill.pdf

Legislation

The following legislation can be viewed in full at www.legislation.gov.uk:

Corporate Manslaughter and Corporate Homicide Act 2007

Health and Safety (Safety Signs and Signals) Regulations 1996

Highway Code 2007

Motorways Traffic (England and Wales) Regulations 1982

Road Safety Act 2006

Road Traffic Act 1988
    Section 36 Road Traffic Act 1988

Road Traffic Exemptions (Special Forces) (Variation and Amendment) Regulations 2011

Road Vehicles (Construction and Use) Regulations 1986
    Regulation 99
    Regulation 107
    Regulation 101

Road Vehicles (Construction and Use) (Amendment No. 2) Regulations 2005

Road Vehicles (Construction and Use) (Amendment No. 4) Regulations 2009

Road Vehicles Lighting (Amendment) Regulations 2005

Road Vehicles Lighting and Goods Vehicles (Plating and Testing) (Amendment) Regulations 2009

Road Vehicles Lighting Regulations 1989
   Regulation 24

Section 62 of the Control of Pollution Act 1974

Section 5 & 87 of the Road Traffic Regulation Act 1984

Serious Organised Crime and Police Act 2005 (Consequential and Supplementary Amendments to Secondary Legislation) Order 2006

Traffic Signs and General Directions Regulations 2002
   Regulations 10 and 26
   Regulation 15(2)
   Regulation 26(5)(b)
   Regulation 27(3)(c)
   Regulations 33, 34, 35, 36(1)(a), 38(a/b)
   Regulation 36(1)(b) (red light)
   Regulations 47, 48, 49

www.gov.uk   (search for 'driver and vehicle licensing')

www.gov.uk   (search for 'medical standards of fitness to drive')

Index

driver characteristics 23
driver competencies 3
driving commentary 22, 110–115
    spot commentaries 113
    system commentary 112–115
driving response system 22
driving skills 22–23
dual carriageways 87
    see also motorways
dynamic risk assessments 22, 92, 98, 99
eco-driving 103–105
electrical systems 66–67
electrical umbilical leads 66–67
electronic brakeforce distribution (EBD) 63, 68
electronic stability programme (ESP) 65–66, 68
emergency start button 66
engine running 11
equipment check 36
exemptions, legal 3, 9, 10–17

fend-off position 94–95
five-phases system of car control 112–113
fuel-efficient driving *see* eco-driving

gearbox
    automatic vehicle 42, 51–60
    familiarisation 41–42
    manual vehicle 41

handbrake test 44–45
hazard warning lights 12, 82, 99
Hazardous Area Response Team (HART) 74
hazards
    anticipation 22, 28, 58, 104, 113

car control system 112–113
driving commentary 111–112, 113–115
fend-off position 94–95
gear selection 59–60
motorways and multi-lane carriageways 89–95
overtaking 55
reversing and manoeuvring 82–85
roadworks 17
slippery road surfaces 65–66
steep gradients 54, 55, 57, 59
High Dependency Service (HDS) vehicles 95, 107, 108
Highway Code 1, 2, 82, 112
Highways Agency Traffic Officers (HATOs) 108–110
horns 17, 35

instructor competencies 3
insurance 4
isolators 67

keep left/right signs 10, 15
key fob 62

laws in relation to driving 1–8, 77–79, 125–126
legal exemptions 3, 9, 10–17
licences
    categories 5–6
    lost/stolen 7
    medical fitness to drive 6, 7
    renewal 6–7, 8
lights
    emergency lighting controls 67–68
    hazard warning lights 12, 82, 99

lighting checks 34
lighting regulations 77–79
warning (flashing) lights
72–73, 75, 78, 99
loading a patient 28, 99

manoeuvring *see* reversing and
manoeuvring
mirrors 39–41
motoring convictions 4
motorways
attending incidents 15–16,
89–97, 107–108
blockage or closure 90–91
motorway regulations 15–16
parking 92–95, 107–108
'Smart Motorways' system 16
travelling in convoy 92
multi-lane carriageways 87, 89
see also motorways

NHS operational fleet 23
no entry signs 18
non-exemptions 9, 17–18

officers' cars 95, 107, 108
one-way signs 18
operational driving stress 24–26
combating 26
professional support 26
overtaking 54, 55, 59

parking
fend-off position 94–95, 107
gear selection 52
legal exemptions 11–12
motorways 92–95, 107–108
non-exemptions 18
urban and rural roads 98–100
passenger comfort 27–28

patient
loading 28, 99
passenger comfort 27–28
Patient Transport Service (PTS)
vehicles 95, 107, 108
pedestrian crossings 11, 14
pedestrian precincts 17
penalty points 4
personal protective equipment
(PPE) 89, 99
police 91, 108
police escorts 100–101
pre-driving check (PDC) 37–48

radio data system (RDS) 74
red mist 12, 13, 98
reversing and manoeuvring
gear selection 52
Highway Code rules and advice
82
reverse sensors 84
teamwork 82–85
Road Safety Act 2006 1, 3
roadworks 17
run lock systems 66

seat belts 18, 46–47
seat position 38–39
sentences for dangerous driving 4
sirens 73, 74, 75
activation 68
situation report (SITREP) 96–97,
98
skidding 65
slippery road surfaces 65–66
'Smart Motorways' system 16
solo responders 75, 99, 101
speed
appropriate 13
eco-driving 104

and safety 115–117
speed limits
exceeding 3, 10, 12–13
legal exemption 3, 10, 12–13
starting the vehicle 42–43
steep gradients 54, 55, 57, 59
stop/give way signs 18
stress *see* operational driving stress

theft of the vehicle, attempted 66
traction control systems 65–66
traffic lights 10, 14
non-exemptions 18

vehicle checks
pre-driving check (PDC)
37–48

vehicle daily inspection (VDI)
32–36
visual warnings
active 72–73, 94
passive 72

warning equipment
dashboard warning signals 63,
68
see also audible warnings; visual
warnings
wheel and tyre checks 33
white lines 11
crossing/straddling 18, 114
windscreen checks 35
work-related stress 25